The Metabolic Management of the Critically Ill

REVIEWING SURGICAL TOPICS

Series Editors: **Thomas King, M.D. and Keith Reemtsma, M.D.**
*Columbia University College of Physicians and Surgeons
New York, New York*

THE METABOLIC MANAGEMENT OF THE CRITICALLY ILL
Douglas W. Wilmore, M.D.

The Metabolic Management of the Critically Ill

Douglas W. Wilmore, M. D.

U. S. Army Institute of Surgical Research
Brooke Army Medical Center
Fort Sam Houston, Texas

PLENUM MEDICAL BOOK COMPANY
New York and London

Library of Congress Cataloging in Publication Data

Wilmore, Douglas W
  The metabolic management of the critically ill.

  (Reviewing surgical topics)
  Includes bibliographical references and index.
  1. Diet in disease. 2. Critically ill. 3. Metabolism. 4. Malnutrition. I.
Title. II. Series.
RM217.W52   616'.025   77-22742

ISBN 978-1-4684-2384-6   ISBN 978-1-4684-2382-2 (eBook)
DOI 10.1007/978-1-4684-2382-2

© 1977 Plenum Publishing Corporation
Softcover reprint of the hardcover 1st edition 1977

227 West 17th Street, New York, N.Y. 10011

Plenum Medical Book Company is an imprint of Plenum Publishing Corporation

Foreword

HOW DO I USE THIS BOOK?

This book is organized to answer specific questions about the metabolic and nutritional problems of critically ill patients. The questions are listed under five chapter headings in the Contents. Each question is self-contained with its own charts, tables, and references, although, in some instances, you may be referred to another section of the book for additional information. A detailed subject outline appears on the first page of each chapter, and there is an index for cross-reference to specific subjects.

A metabolic support plan and accompanying metabolic and nutritional worksheet are located in the Appendix. This plan provides the best estimates available for predicting the metabolic requirements of patients, and outlines approaches to feeding the hospitalized patient which will satisfy these nutritional needs. Clinical cases are presented in this section to help you get started using the support plan.

This volume is a handbook organized for frequent use — place the appropriate tables and nomograms on the bulletin board of the intensive care unit or in your office for convenient reference. Use the metabolic and nutritional support plan and establish the habit of assessing the metabolic requirements of your patients. Refer to the references cited to explore in further detail specific questions or areas of interest. By applying our knowledge of the metabolic and nutritional alterations which occur following disease, we can improve our care of the critically ill.

Contents

A detailed outline of subjects appears on the first page of each seotion

CHAPTER 1

Energy and Energy Balance

1.1 WHAT IS THE BODY'S EFFICIENCY IN CONVERTING CHEMICAL ENERGY INTO MECHANICAL WORK? WHAT IS THE EFFICIENCY IN ENERGY CONVERSION TO HEAT?

Man is an energy machine able to convert food or body fuel stores to mechanical work. The efficiency of energy conversion to work can be calculated from the ratio of external work to internal energy

1

conversion rate. In fed man, a small portion of heat is lost following the intake of food, and this is called the entropy or free energy of a foodstuff, indicating that part of the energy obtained from food is thermodynamically obligated for conversion to heat. This may account for 5–10% of the initial heat lost. The conversion of food energy into high-energy biochemical bonds is inefficient, and about half of the potential energy from food is dissipated as heat. Of the remaining 45% of the free-energy pool stored as ATP or other high-energy bonds, only about half is utilized for external work,

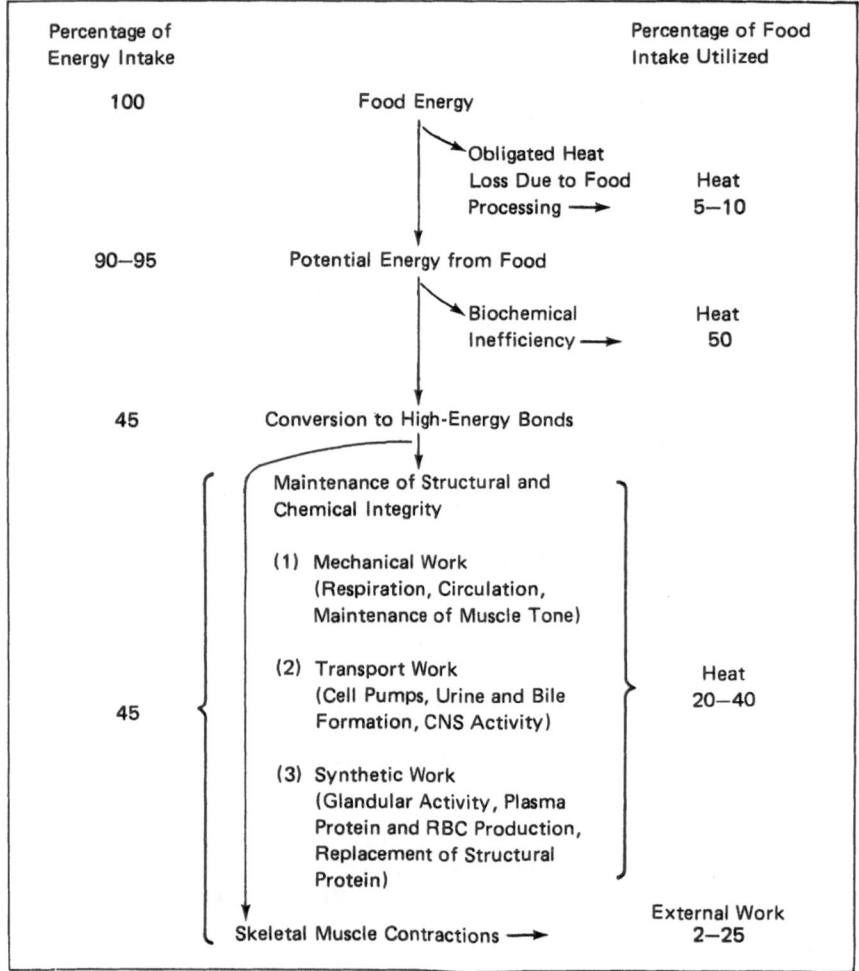

FIGURE 1.1: The conversion of food energy to heat and work.

which occurs only when skeletal muscles are used. The majority of high-energy substances are utilized for internal work (respiration, circulation, cell pumps, etc.), resulting in the generation of a large quantity of heat (Fig. 1.1).

Chemical energy derived from food or body fuels is distributed between heat and work. At maximum efficiency, about 25% of chemical energy is converted to mechanical work, the remainder to heat. At rest, almost all oxidized energy may be accounted for by heat lost from the body. Thus, the efficiency for the body at rest to convert fuel to heat is almost 100%. The energy utilized in hospitalized patients is almost totally reflected in heat lost from the body.

1.2   WHAT IS A KILOCALORIE?

A calorie is the amount of heat required to raise the temperature of 1 g of water from 14.5° to 15.5°C at a pressure of one standard atmosphere. A calorie is often written as "$cal_{15°}$," and is also referred to as a gram-calorie. A kilocalorie (kcal) is 1000 calories, and is the traditional measure used in clinical nutrition in this country to refer to units of energy. A kilocalorie was once referred to as a "large" or "big" calorie, but this form is infrequently used. Other units of energy are referred to in countries where the metric system is utilized: the joule (J) is the unit of energy agreed on by the International System of Units and the watt (W) is the unit of power (energy per unit time). The conversion factors for these units are:

$$1 \text{ kilocalorie (kcal}_{15°}) = 4.186 \text{ kilojoule (kJ)}[1]$$
$$1 \text{ joule/sec} = 1 \text{ watt (W)}$$
$$1 \text{ kilocalorie} = 1.16 \text{ watt hours (Wh)}$$

Tables 1.1 and 1.2 demonstrate use of these conversion factors.

---

[1] There are three different factors for converting calories to joules, depending on the type of calorie utilized: the thermochemical calorie, 15° calorie, or the International Steam Table calorie. Interested readers are referred to Kleiber's delightful discussion of the complex problem of energy units and conversion factors (Kleiber, M.: Joules vs. calories in nutrition. *J. Nutr., 102*:309, 1972).

Table 1.1   Energy Equivalents

Kilocalories kcal	Kilojoules kJ	Watt hours Wh	Kilocalories kcal	Kilojoules kJ	Watt hours Wh
1	4.180	1.160	36	150.480	41.760
2	8.360	2.320	37	154.660	42.920
3	12.540	3.480	38	158.840	44.080
4	16.720	4.640	39	163.020	45.240
5	20.900	5.800	40	167.200	46.400
6	25.080	6.960	41	171.380	47.560
7	29.260	8.120	42	175.560	48.720
8	33.440	9.280	43.	179.740	49.880
9	37.620	10.440	44	183.920	51.040
10	41.800	11.600	45	188.100	52.200
11	45.980	12.760	46.	192.280	53.360
12	50.160	13.920	47	196.460	54.520
13	54.340	15.080	48	200.640	55.680
14	58.520	16.240	49	204.820	56.840
15	62.700	17.400	50	209.000	58.000
16	66.880	18.560	51	213.180	59.160
17	71.060	19.720	52	217.360	60.320
18	75.240	20.880	53	221.540	61.480
19	79.420	22.040	54	225.720	62.640
20	83.600	23.200	55	229.900	63.800
21	87.780	24.360	56	234.080	64.960
22	91.960	25.520	57	238.260	66.120
23	96.140	26.680	58	242.440	67.280
24	100.320	27.840	59	246.620	68.440
25	104.500	29.000	60	250.800	69.600
26	108.680	30.160	61	254.980	70.760
27	112.860	31.320	62	259.160	71.920
28	117.040	32.480	63.	263.340	73.080
29	121.220	33.640	64	267.520	74.240
30	125.400	34.800	65	271.700	75.400
31	129.580	35.960	66	275.880	76.560
32	133.760	37.120	67	280.060	77.720
33	137.940	38.280	68	284.240	78.880
34	142.120	39.440	69	288.420	80.040
35	146.300	40.600	70	292.600	81.200

Table 1.1 — continued

Kilocalories kcal	Kilojoules kJ	Watt hours Wh	Kilocalories kcal	Kilojoules kJ	Watt hours Wh
71	296.780	82.360	700	2926.000	812.000
72	300.960	83.520	800	3344.000	928.000
73	305.140	84.680	900	3762.000	1044.000
74	309.320	85.840	1000	4180.000	1160.000
75	313.500	87.000	1100	4598.000	1276.000
76	317.680	88.160	1200	5016.000	1392.000
77	321.860	89.320	1300	5434.000	1508.000
78	326.040	90.480	1400	5852.000	1624.000
79	330.220	91.640	1500	6270.000	1740.000
80	334.400	92.800	1600	6688.000	1856.000
81	338.580	93.960	1700	7106.000	1972.000
82	342.760	95.120	1800	7524.000	2088.000
83	346.940	96.280	1900	7942.000	2204.000
84	351.120	97.440	2000	8360.000	2320.000
85	355.300	98.600	2100	8778.000	2436.000
86	359.480	99.760	2200	9196.000	2552.000
87	363.660	100.920	2300	9614.000	2668.000
88	367.840	102.080	2400	10032.000	2784.000
89	372.020	103.240	2500	10450.000	2900.000
90	376.200	104.400	2600	10868.000	3016.000
91	380.380	105.560	2700	11286.000	3132.000
92	384.560	106.720	2800	11704.000	3248.000
93	388.740	107.880	2900	12121.999	3364.000
94	392.920	109.040	3000	12539.999	3480.000
95	397.100	110.200	3100	12957.999	3596.000
96	401.280	111.360	3200	13375.999	3712.000
97	405.460	112.520	3300	13793.999	3828.000
98	409.640	113.680	3400	14211.999	3944.000
99	413.820	114.840	3500	14629.999	4060.000
100	418.000	116.000	3600	15047.999	4176.000
200	836.000	232.000	3700	15465.999	4292.000
300	1254.000	348.000	3800	15883.999	4408.000
400	1672.000	464.000	3900	16301.999	4524.000
500	2090.000	580.000	4000	16720.000	4640.000
600	2508.000	696.000			

Table   1.2   Examples   of   Energy   Expenditure   Using
Various Energy Units

Rate of energy expenditure (70 kg man)			
	O_2 (ml/min)	kcal/min	kJ/min	W
Sitting	250	1.2	5.0	84
Walking	1000	4.8	20.1	334
Exertion	5000	24.2	101.2	1684

Food conversions			
	kcal	kJ	Wh
1 g carbohydrate	4	16.7	4.6
1 g fat	9	37.6	10.4
1 g protein	4	16.7	4.6

Energy content of diets			
	kcal	MJ	Wh
Reducing	1000	4.2	1160
Maintenance (sedentary individual)	2500	10.4	2900
Maintenance (heavy work load)	3300	13.8	3828

1.3   WHAT IS THERMAL BALANCE?

Energy can be neither created nor destroyed; hence the energy or heat produced by the body can be accounted for as heat lost and/or stored in the body:

$$\text{Heat produced} = \text{Heat lost} + \text{Heat stored}$$

Heat storage is a process in which the heat produced by the body is retained in body tissues, causing an alteration in mean body temperature. For example, an individual exercising on a hot day does not lose all the heat he produces and his core temperature rises as he stores heat. After exercise, the additional heat stored in the body dissipates and core temperature returns slowly to normal. Negative heat storage would be associated with a fall in mean body temperature.

Because man is a homotherm and maintains a relatively stable body temperature within narrow limits, heat storage or loss does not usually occur in the steady state, and heat production can be equated with heat loss. That is:

$$\text{Heat produced} = \text{Heat lost}[2]$$

1.4 HOW IS HEAT LOSS FROM THE BODY MEASURED? WHAT IS DIRECT CALORIMETRY?

Calorimetry is the measurement of energy expenditure. Heat lost from the body may be measured directly by whole-body or direct calorimetry. The subject is placed in a sealed, insulated, boxlike chamber, the temperature across the walls maintained at a constant level, and heat produced by the subject is removed from the chamber by water circulating through the coils which are inside the chamber. The rate of dry heat transfer from the individual to the coils is computed from the increase in water temperature and the rate of water flowing through the coils. Air is circulated through the chamber and its water vapor analyzed to determine wet heat loss (Fig. 1.2).

The use of a chamber for direct calorimetry is an arduous and slow process.[3] The patient should be in a steady state and at equilibrium with the walls of the chamber. Because the chamber is small, the environment within the compartment may change if not carefully controlled. These problems have been resolved in part by the development of gradient layer calorimeters for direct measurement of heat loss from the body. When heat is transmitted across a layer of thermally conducting matter, a difference in temperature exists between the surfaces of the layer. Thermocouples are placed on the inside and outside of the insulated surfaces of the calorimeter. By knowing the temperature of the surfaces and the thermo-conductivity of the layer, heat loss from an object in the calorimeter is determined. The temperature measurements are made instantaneously, summed, and continuously recorded. Small gradient layer calorimeters are available for animal research, and large calorimeters,

---

[2]Mean body temperature unchanged.

[3]Coleman, W., and DuBois, E. F.: Clinical calorimetry. VII; Calorimetric observations on the metabolism of typhoid patients with and without food. *Arch. Intern. Med.*, 15:887, 1915.

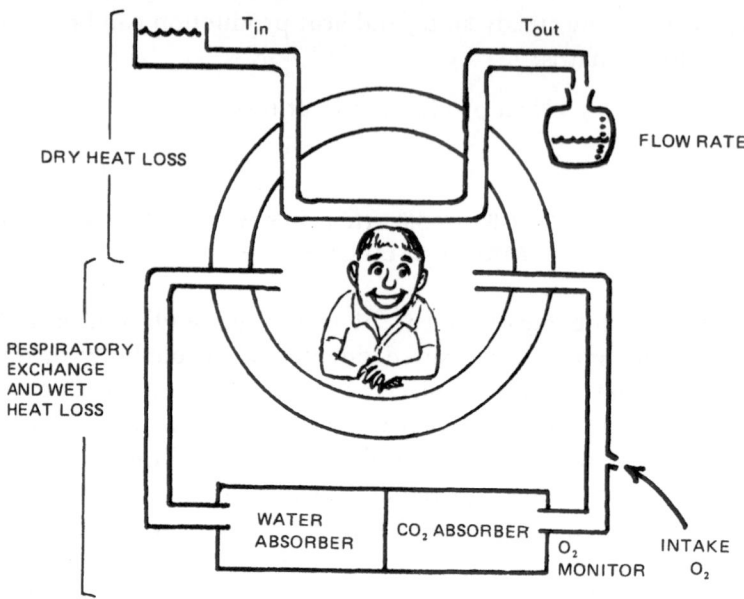

FIGURE 1.2: One method of direct calorimetry.

containing thousands of thermocouples, have been utilized to
measure heat loss in man.[4]

In clinical medicine, however, these techniques are rarely
employed to determine heat loss or heat production; rather, indirect
calorimetry is the method preferred.

1.5   WHAT IS INDIRECT CALORIMETRY?

In the steady state, oxygen consumed and carbon dioxide produced
are related to the release of energy from the body. The relationship
between energy release and the quantity of these two gases is
stoichiometric for any particular reaction, although the gas exchange
for all foodstuffs is not the same. For example, the oxidation of
glucose yields the following reaction:

$$C_6H_{12}O_6 + 6\,O_2 = 6\,H_2O + 6\,CO_2 + 673 \text{ kcal}$$

[4]Bradham, G. B.: Direct measurement of total metabolism of a burn patient. *Arch. Surg.,*
105:410, 1972.

A constant amount of oxygen is consumed, and a constant amount of carbon dioxide is produced for each mole of glucose oxidized. We can measure the heat generated by this reaction directly (in a direct or bomb calorimeter), or we can quantitate the amount of oxygen consumed and carbon dioxide produced and relate these gas volumes to heat production. Measurement of gas exchange is the basis of the technique of indirect calorimetry.

The classic studies by Atwater and Benedict[5] demonstrated the close correlation between measurements of heat production in man using direct and indirect techniques. As a result, indirect calorimetry (based on gas exchange of the individual) has become an accepted method for determining the rate of energy expenditure.

1.6   HOW IS OXYGEN CONSUMPTION RELATED TO HEAT PRODUCTION?

In a resting subject who consumes an average American diet, studied in the postabsorptive state, 4.83 kcal are generated for every liter of oxygen consumed. That is:

$$\text{Metabolic rate} = 4.83 \times \dot{V}_{O_2}$$

Not all foodstuffs utilize the same amount of oxygen (see Table 1.3), but this estimate will determine heat production within approximately 8% of the true value no matter which nutrient is being oxidized (the largest error occurs with the oxidation of protein).

1.7   HOW MUCH OXYGEN IS CONSUMED BY NORMAL MAN? HOW DOES OXYGEN CONSUMPTION AFFECT RESPIRATION?

Heat loss in the idealized "normal man" (1.73 m^2, 70 kg body weight) is about 60—70 kcal/hr. This quantity of heat will require the consumption of 12.5—14.5 liters of oxygen/hr, or approximately 210—250 ml oxygen consumed/min. The amount of air that a normal man should breathe (resting minute ventilation) is

[5]Atwater, W. O., and Benedict, F. G.: Experiments on the metabolism of matter and energy in the human body. *USDA Office of Experimental Stations Bulletin Publication No. 136*, 1903.

Table 1.3   The Energy and Respiratory Equivalent of Body Fuels

Food	Energy (kcal/g)		Respiratory equivalent			Volume	
	Bomb calorimeter	Human oxidation	Physiological value	O_2 (kcal/liter)	CO_2 (kcal/liter)	R.Q. ($\dot{V}CO_2/\dot{V}O_2$)	O_2 (liter/g)	CO_2 (liter/g)
Carbohydrate	4.1	4.1	4	5.05	5.05	1.00	0.81	0.81
Protein[a]	5.4	4.2	4	4.46	5.57	0.80	0.94	0.75
Fat	9.3	9.3	9	4.74	6.67	0.71	1.96	1.39
Alcohol	7.1	7.1	7	4.86	7.25	0.67	1.46	0.98
Average				4.83	5.89	0.82		

[a]Protein oxidation exclusive of nitrogen and sulfa excreted in urine.

(Adapted from: Brown, A. C.: Energy metabolism, *In* Ruch, T. C., and Patton, H. D. (Eds.): *Physiology and Biophysics III*, Philadelphia, W. B. Saunders, 1973, p. 92.)

determined by his anatomic dead space, tidal volume, and frequency of breathing on one hand and his metabolic requirements on the other. Homeostatic mechanisms provide for adequate oxygen transport across the alveoli while carbon dioxide is exhaled in the expired air to maintain a normal blood pCO_2. This balance is achieved in normal man (70 kg) by breathing approximately 6–7 liters of air/min. At this minute ventilation, only about one-fifth of the inspired oxygen is actually consumed. The oxygen content of the atmosphere is approximately 21%, and decreases to 16–18% in expired air. An increase in oxygen consumption is associated with an increase in minute ventilation and pulse rate, and these two additional measurements have frequently been related to metabolic activity, especially in exercising man.[6] Minute ventilation and pulse rate are useful bedside determinants of energy expenditure in patients with normal cardiorespiratory function. However, they become less useful correlates with heat production in patients with respiratory or cardiac failure.

1.8 WHAT DOES TOTAL BODY OXYGEN CONSUMPTION MEASURE?

Measurement of oxygen consumption reflects the sum of the oxygen consumed by various organ systems of the body. At rest, liver, skeletal muscle, and brain contribute the greatest proportion of heat produced during the basal state (Table 1.4). During exercise, the proportion of oxygen consumed by the skeletal muscles greatly increases and this elevation is related to the extent of the exercise. Although the exact proportion of organ heat production is not known in infected or injured patients, our studies suggest that liver and skeletal muscle are the greatest contributors to this increased heat load.

1.9 HOW IS OXYGEN CONSUMPTION MEASURED?

The most frequent methods for measurement of oxygen consumption are by closed-circuit or open-circuit techniques. The closed-circuit method utilizes a spirometer, which is filled with oxygen or

---

[6]Datta, S. R., and Ramanathan, N. L.: Energy expenditure in work predicted from heart rate and pulmonary ventilation. *J. Appl. Physiol.*, 26:297, 1969.

Table 1.4   Organ Oxygen Consumption[a]

Organ	Weight (kg)	% of body weight	Oxygen consumption		% of basal metabolism
			Per kg (ml/min)	Whole organ (ml/min)	
Liver	1.5	2.1	44	66	26.4
Brain	1.4	2.0	33	46	18.3
Heart	0.3	0.43	94	23	9.2
Kidneys	0.3	0.43	61	18	7.2
Skeletal muscle	27.8	39.7	2.3	64	25.6
Total				217	86.7

[a]From: Brožek, J., and Grande, F.: Body composition and basal metabolism in man: correlation analysis versus physiological approach. *Hum. Biol.,* 27:22, 1955.

room air. A carbon dioxide absorber is placed in the circuit and the subject breathes from the spirometer through a mouthpiece, after a nose clip or nose plugs have been applied. Alternately, a face mask may be employed to interface with the apparatus. With inspiration, gas flows from the spirometer into the lungs, and a portion of the oxygen is utilized. The carbon dioxide produced is removed by the CO_2 absorber, and the remainder of the expired gas returns to the spirometer. The volume decrease of the spirometer over a measured period of time represents the rate of oxygen consumed (Fig. 1.3).

The open-circuit method utilizes a set of one-way valves to direct expired air into a collecting container (usually Douglas bags or a Tissot spirometer, although a modification of this technique has been employed utilizing a canopy hood). At the end of a carefully timed collecting period, both the volume and composition of the expired air are measured and the rate of oxygen consumption and carbon dioxide production determined by the difference between the concentrations of outside air and the gas collected:

20.9 (outside air O_2) — Bag O_2 concentration

$$= \text{Volume } \% \ O_2 \text{ extracted}$$

$$\frac{\text{Volume gas moved}}{\text{Unit time}} \times \frac{\text{Volume } \% \ O_2 \text{ consumed}}{\text{Unit time}} = \frac{O_2 \text{ consumption}}{\text{Unit time}}$$

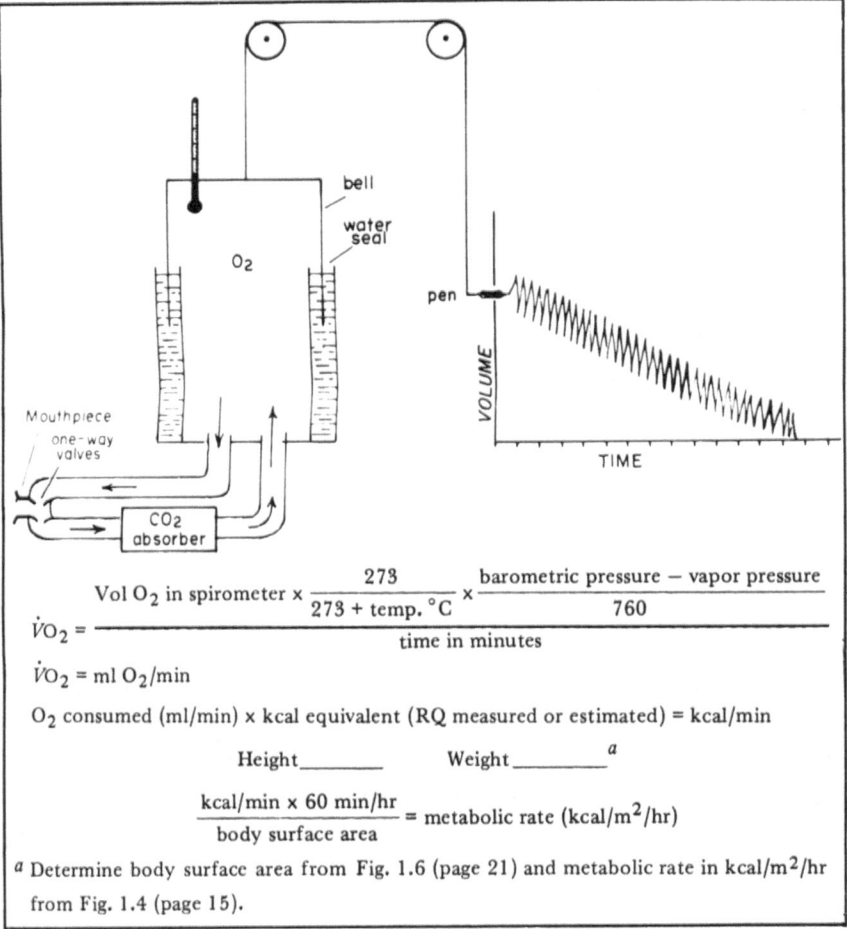

$$\dot{V}O_2 = \frac{\text{Vol } O_2 \text{ in spirometer} \times \dfrac{273}{273 + \text{temp. } °C} \times \dfrac{\text{barometric pressure} - \text{vapor pressure}}{760}}{\text{time in minutes}}$$

$\dot{V}O_2$ = ml O_2/min

O_2 consumed (ml/min) × kcal equivalent (RQ measured or estimated) = kcal/min

Height_____   Weight_____[a]

$$\frac{\text{kcal/min} \times 60 \text{ min/hr}}{\text{body surface area}} = \text{metabolic rate (kcal/m}^2\text{/hr)}$$

[a] Determine body surface area from Fig. 1.6 (page 21) and metabolic rate in kcal/m²/hr from Fig. 1.4 (page 15).

FIGURE 1.3: Data sheet for calculation of oxygen consumption from a spirometer (closed system).

0 (outside CO_2) + Bag CO_2 concentration

= Volume CO_2 % produced

$$\frac{\text{Volume gas moved}}{\text{Unit time}} \times \frac{\text{Volume \% } CO_2 \text{ produced}}{\text{Unit time}} = \frac{CO_2 \text{ production}}{\text{Unit time}}$$

These volumes must be corrected because of the small difference which occurs between the volume of inspired and expired gas, accounted for by the discrepancy of volumes between oxygen consumed and carbon dioxide produced. Finally, the gas volume is corrected for standard temperature and pressure and dry gas concentrations so that all measurements are equated with 0°C, 760 mm Hg barometric pressure and dry gas.

The volumes measured per unit time may then be converted to energy equivalents by the following equation:

$$\text{Heat/unit time} = 3.9 \dot{V}_{O_2} + 1.1 \dot{V}_{CO_2}$$

or

$$\text{Heat/unit time} = \dot{V}_{O_2} (3.9 + 1.1 \text{ respiratory quotient})$$

If urinary nitrogen measurements are included, the formula described by Weir can be utilized:[7]

$$\text{Heat produced/unit time} = 3.94 \dot{V}_{O_2} + 1.11 \dot{V}_{CO_2}$$
$$- 2.17 \text{ urinary nitrogen}$$

1.10   CAN CARBON DIOXIDE PRODUCTION BE EQUATED TO ENERGY PRODUCTION?

Carbon dioxide production has been used by many investigators to measure heat production. Carbon dioxide production is a sensitive indicator of the type of foodstuff metabolized, and hence varies much more than oxygen consumption with the ingested diet. Moreover, the body contains large stores of CO_2, and a decrease in pH or hyperventilation will reduce body CO_2 stores and increase the CO_2 content of the expired air. No method exists for distinguishing this stored CO_2 from that produced by substrate oxidation, and hence the subject would appear hypermetabolic if only CO_2 were used to determine heat production under these conditions. Because of a greater variability in CO_2 production and storage, oxygen is the preferred gas for the determination of metabolic heat production.

1.11   WHAT IS RQ? WHY IS IT USEFUL?

The respiratory quotient or RQ is the ratio of volume of carbon dioxide produced divided by the volume of oxygen consumed during

---

[7]Weir, J. B. deV: New methods for calculating metabolic rate with special reference to protein metabolism. *J. Physiol.*, *109*:1, 1949.

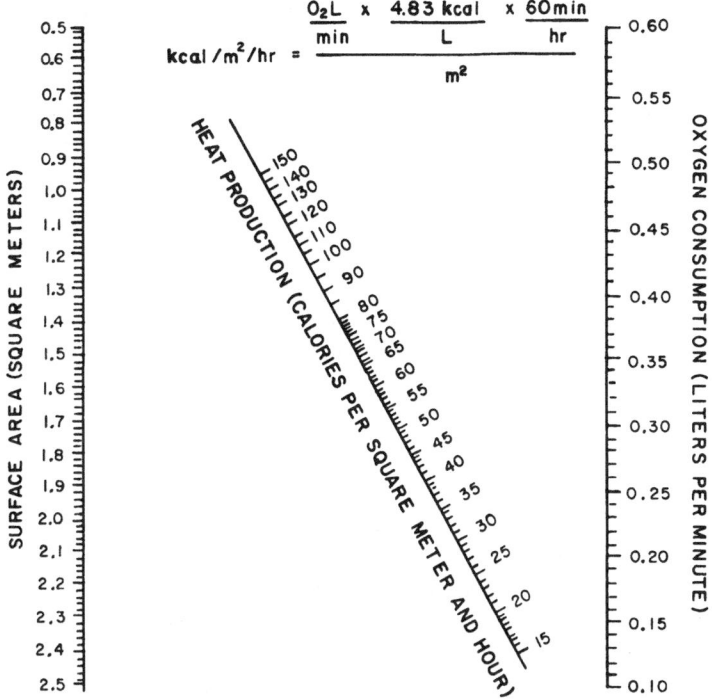

$$kcal/m^2/hr = \frac{\dfrac{O_2L}{min} \times \dfrac{4.83\ kcal}{L} \times \dfrac{60\ min}{hr}}{m^2}$$

FIGURE 1.4: Heat production (kcal/m^2/hr) from surface area and oxygen consumption. Locate body surface area (Fig. 1.6, page 21) on the scale at the left and measured oxygen consumption (liters/min) on the right-hand scale. Connecting the two points with a straightedge will determine metabolic activity (assuming an RQ of 0.82).

the same time period ($\dot{V}CO_2/\dot{V}O_2$). Normally, RQ ranges between 0.70 and 1.00 and varies with substrate oxidation (Table 1.5). The usual subject on a typical diet, studied several hours after the ingestion of food, will have a measured RQ between 0.80 and 0.85. RQ will decrease toward 0.70 with prolonged fasting, demonstrating the almost complete fat oxidation during the starved state. Hyperventilation increases the RQ, often above 1, and this reflects a nonsteady state and inaccurate test situation. The RQ moves toward 1 with dietary carbohydrate loading and, if carbohydrate is converted to fat (that is, when carbohydrate intake exceeds metabolic requirements), the RQ may exceed 1 (Table 1.5). Although RQs below 0.70 have been associated with oxidation of ketones or synthesis of carbohydrate from fat, values below 0.70 should be

Table 1.5   Mean Respiratory Gases Measured During Three Levels of Feeding
in Six Critically Ill Patients

Calorie intake	600 kcal/day	3000 kcal/day	6000 kcal/day
$\dot{V}CO_2$ (ml/min)	259	302	345
$\dot{V}O_2$ (ml/min)	325	337	341
RQ	0.80	0.89	1.01

Adapted from: Wilmore, D. W., Curreri, P. W., Spitzer, K. W., Spitzer, M. E., and Pruitt, B.
A., Jr.: Supranormal dietary intake in thermally injured patients. *Surg. Gynecol. Obstet.*,
132:881, 1971.

regarded with great skepticism, for they usually reflect methodological error.

RQ provides a general indicator of the nature of body
metabolism, and reflects methodological error in gas collection and
measurement. Respiratory gas also reflects the oxygen consumption
and carbon dioxide production yielded from protein metabolism.
With the combustion of the quantity of protein which produces 1 g
urinary nitrogen, 5.94 liters of O_2 are consumed and 4.76 liters of
CO_2 are produced. A timed urine collection (usually over at least
2 hr) is made and urinary nitrogen excretion determined. The
contribution of protein combustion to gas exchange may be
calculated, and this correction in total gas exchange will yield the
"nonprotein RQ".[8] The calculations by the Weir equation for
determining total heat production corrects for the nitrogen contribution by assuming that 12.5% of the total oxidized calories arise
from protein production. The error generated by not including
urinary nitrogen excretion in the calculation of heat production is
usually less than 2%.

1.12   HOW IS THE FUEL SOURCE OF THE ENERGY OXIDIZED BY THE BODY DETERMINED?

As previously noted, RQ provides a general indicator of the nature of
the body fuel metabolized. RQ values between 0.7 and 1.0 reflect

[8]Peters, J. P., and Van Slyke, D. D.: *Quantitative Clinical Chemistry*, Vol. II. Baltimore,
Williams and Wilkins, 1932, p. 207.

Table 1.6   Worksheet for Calculation of Substrate Oxidation, Metabolic Water, and Heat Production (All Standardized per Unit Time)

	Urinary nitrogen (grams)	Oxygen consumed (liters)	Carbon dioxide (liters)	Sum of values
Protein (g)	+6.25 x ____			
Carbohydrate (g)	−2.56 x ____	−2.91 x ____	+4.12 x ____	= ____
Fat (g)	−1.94 x ____	+1.69 x ____	−1.69 x ____	= ____
Metabolic water (g)	−1.04 x ____	+0.062 x ____	+0.662 x ____	= ____
Metabolic heat (kcal)	−2.98 x ____	+3.78 x ____	+1.16 x ____	= ____

These equations were derived from the following formulas:

$\dot{V}O_2$ = 6.03 nitrogen in the urine + 0.83 carbohydrate in the diet + 2.02 fat in the diet.

$\dot{V}CO_2$ = 4.88 nitrogen in the urine + 0.829 carbohydrate in the diet + 1.43 fat in the diet.

Adapted from: Consolazio, C. F., Johnson, R. E., and Pecora, L. J.: *Physiological Measurements of Metabolic Functions in Man.* New York, McGraw-Hill, 1963, p. 316.

varying percentage of fat and carbohydrate being oxidized, with protein metabolism quantitated by the amount of urinary nitrogen excreted. Many of the formulas that calculate heat production from oxygen consumption and carbon dioxide production have accounted for the carbon loss due to protein catabolism. However, by measuring urinary nitrogen, protein metabolism can be accounted for by the nitrogen residue broken down from amino acids and incorporated into urea which is excreted in the urine. Measurement of oxygen consumption, carbon dioxide production, and urinary nitrogen allows determination of individual fuel sources oxidized as well as calculation of the total quantity of heat produced. A worksheet for calculation of metabolic oxidation is provided; all units should be expressed for the same time period.

1.13   WHAT IS BMR? WHAT IS RME?

Basal metabolic rate is the measured rate of heat production compared with a predicted standard:

$$BMR = \frac{\text{Measured kcal} - \text{Predicted kcal}}{\text{Predicted kcal}} \times 100$$

BMR is expressed as a positive or negative percentage factor of normal, and a range of ±10−12 is generally accepted as the normal variation in measurement when compared with the predicted normal value.[9] Standards may be obtained from previously determined measurements available from tables,[10] nomograms, or equations.[11]

Clinicians have frequently referred to the standards of Boothby and associates[10] or to the Harris–Benedict equation for calculation of standard basal metabolic rate.[11] These standards are slightly high and represent the results of test results from untrained subjects. Repeated measurements taken over several consecutive days demonstrate a decrease in metabolic rate of 8–9% with training. We have utilized the standards suggested by Fleisch,[12] who calculated metabolic rate in kcal/m^2/hr from 24 sets of published standards. These values are approximately 8% below the standards of Boothby but represent the best standards available to the clinician.

Measurement of basal metabolic rate should be performed under carefully controlled circumstances. The fasting, rested subject is studied in the early morning in a darkened, quiet room while completely at rest and in the recumbent position. Such circumstances in critically ill patients are frequently impossible because of the treatment and care required, yet measurement of energy requirements is important to determine caloric needs and the intake necessary to attain positive energy balance. Metabolic rate measured in the critically ill patient is often referred to as "resting metabolic expenditure" because of the difficulties in controlling all conditions during gas exchange measurements. RME describes the energy needed by a hospitalized patient and usually includes the BMR plus energy required for eating and minimal physical activity. However, even these measurements should be performed under controlled defined conditions in order to interpret the results.

Finally, anxiety may elevate the rate of oxygen consumption. The test should be performed in duplicate or triplicate with rest periods between the measurements. This helps to acquaint the subject with the apparatus, allays anxiety, and usually provides a satisfactory reproducible measurement by the second or third test.

[9]DuBois, E.: *Basal Metabolism in Health and Disease.* New York, Lea and Febiger, 1924.
[10]Boothby, W. M., Berkson, J., and Dunn, H. L.: Studies of the energy metabolism of normal individuals. *Amer. J. Physiol.,* 116:468, 1936.
[11]Harris, J. A., and Benedict, F. G.: Biometric studies of basal metabolism in man. *Carnegie Institution of Washington, Publication No. 279,* 1919.
[12]Fleisch, A.: Le metabolisme basal standard et sa determination au moyen du "Metabocalculator." *Helv. Med. Acta, 18:*23, 1951.

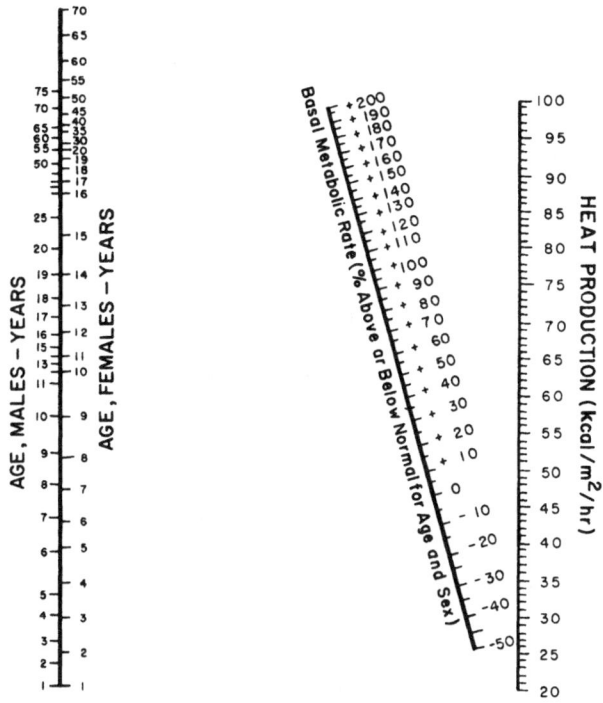

FIGURE 1.5: Basal metabolic rate from heat production, age, and sex. Basal metabolic rate is determined by locating age on left-hand scale, measured heat production on right-hand scale, connecting the two points with a straightedge, and reading BMR on the middle scale.

1.14   HOW DOES BODY SIZE AFFECT METABOLIC RATE? HOW DO WE CORRECT FOR BODY WEIGHT?

An adult produces more heat per day than a child because of increased cellular mass. Thus, metabolic rate is positively related to body size because a larger collection of cells or larger individual cells require more oxygen for maintenance of functional integrity. To compare metabolic rate, and, more particularly, basal metabolic rates in humans, heat production is generally expressed in kilocalories per square meter body surface area; the heat produced per square meter surface area of an adult can be compared to the heat produced per square meter body surface area of another subject such as a child. This surface law holds true for a wide range of biologic species ranging in body size from the mouse to the cow. This linear relationship is not true if metabolic rate or oxygen consumption is expressed per kilogram body weight. However, Kleiber found that body weight raised to the three-quarter power (or, more precisely, weight in kilograms to the 0.734 power) was related to body surface area,[13] and proposed that the resting metabolic rate (MR) of mammals could be calculated by the following equations:

$$MR \text{ (kcal/day)} = 70 \times \text{weight}^{3/4}$$
$$MR \text{ (kcal/hr)} = 3 \times \text{weight}^{3/4}$$
$$\text{Weight} = \text{kg body weight}$$

Because the power conversion is cumbersome, most individuals determine body surface areas from standard height and weight measurements and express heat production in terms of kilocalories per square meter of body surface area per unit time, or oxygen consumption in milliliters per square meter per unit time. Surface area is an acceptable method of comparing heat expenditure of one patient with another and this reference unit may also be used in calculating calorie and nitrogen intake.

The surface area reference, which includes both height and weight, has an additional advantage for the clinician over weight alone or body weight raised to a power. In critically ill patients, short-term alterations in body weight are frequently the result of fluid loss or gain and body weight is therefore not an accurate reflection of body mass under these conditions. This error is minimized by utilizing both height and weight to calculate the reference standard of body surface area.[14]

Techniques for estimating basal metabolic rate in normal individuals are as follows:

A. From height and weight

1. Determine body surface area from the accompanying nomogram (Fig. 1.6).
2. Determine metabolic rate from predicted standards for age and sex of the subject (Table 1.7).

[13]Kleiber, M.: *The Fire of Life — An Introduction to Animal Energetics.* New York, John Wiley, 1961.

[14]Dubois, D., and Dubois, E. F.: Clinical calorimetry: a formula to estimate the approximate surface area if height and weight be known. *Arch. Intern. Med., 17*:863, 1916.

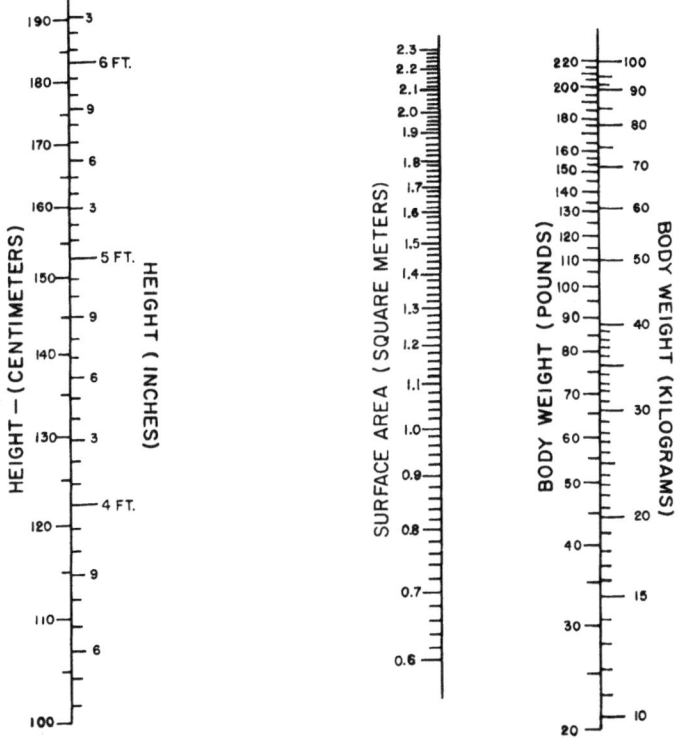

FIGURE 1.6: Surface area from height and weight. To determine body surface area from the height on the left-hand scale and weight on the right-hand scale, connect these points with a straightedge and read surface area from the middle scale.

3. Multiply body surface area times metabolic rate or use accompanying nomogram (Fig. 1.7) for calculation of daily or hourly energy expenditure.

B. From weight alone

   1. For persons of "average" height, use accompanying nomogram (Fig. 1.8) and follow the procedure listed above.
   2. For adults, use $kg^{0.75}$ conversion table (Table 1.8).

1.15 WHY IS METABOLIC RATE RELATED TO BODY SIZE?

In a general sense, the quantity of oxygen consumed per unit time is related to the number and size of the cell population. The

Table 1.7   Standard Metabolic Rates[a]

Age in years	kcal/m²/hr		kJ/m²/hr	
	Men	Women	Men	Women
1	53.0	53.0	222	222
2	52.4	52.4	219	219
3	51.3	51.2	215	214
4	50.3	49.8	211	208
5	49.3	48.4	206	203
6	48.3	47.0	202	197
7	47.3	45.4	198	190
8	46.3	43.8	194	183
9	45.2	42.8	189	179
10	44.0	42.5	184	178
11	43.0	42.0	180	176
12	42.5	41.3	178	173
13	42.3	40.3	177	169
14	42.1	39.2	176	164
15	41.8	37.9	175	159
16	41.4	36.9	173	154
17	40.8	36.3	171	152
18	40.0	35.9	167	150
19	39.2	35.5	164	149
20	38.6	35.3	162	148
25	37.5	35.2	157	147
30	36.8	35.1	154	147
35	36.5	35.0	153	146
40	36.3	34.9	152	146
45	36.2	34.5	152	144
50	35.8	33.9	150	142
55	35.4	33.3	148	139
60	34.9	32.7	146	137
65	34.4	32.2	144	135
70	33.8	31.7	141	133
75 and over	33.2	31.3	139	131

[a]Fleisch, A.: Le metabolisme basal standard et sa determination au moyen du "Metabocalculator," *Helv. Med. Acta, 18:*23, 1951.

relationship was thought to depend on surface area because of the need for heat loss from the body. Alternately, this relationship may be related to the circulatory capacity of the body to nourish the body cell mass and transport heat to the surface for dissipation. Others have related oxygen consumption to lean body mass

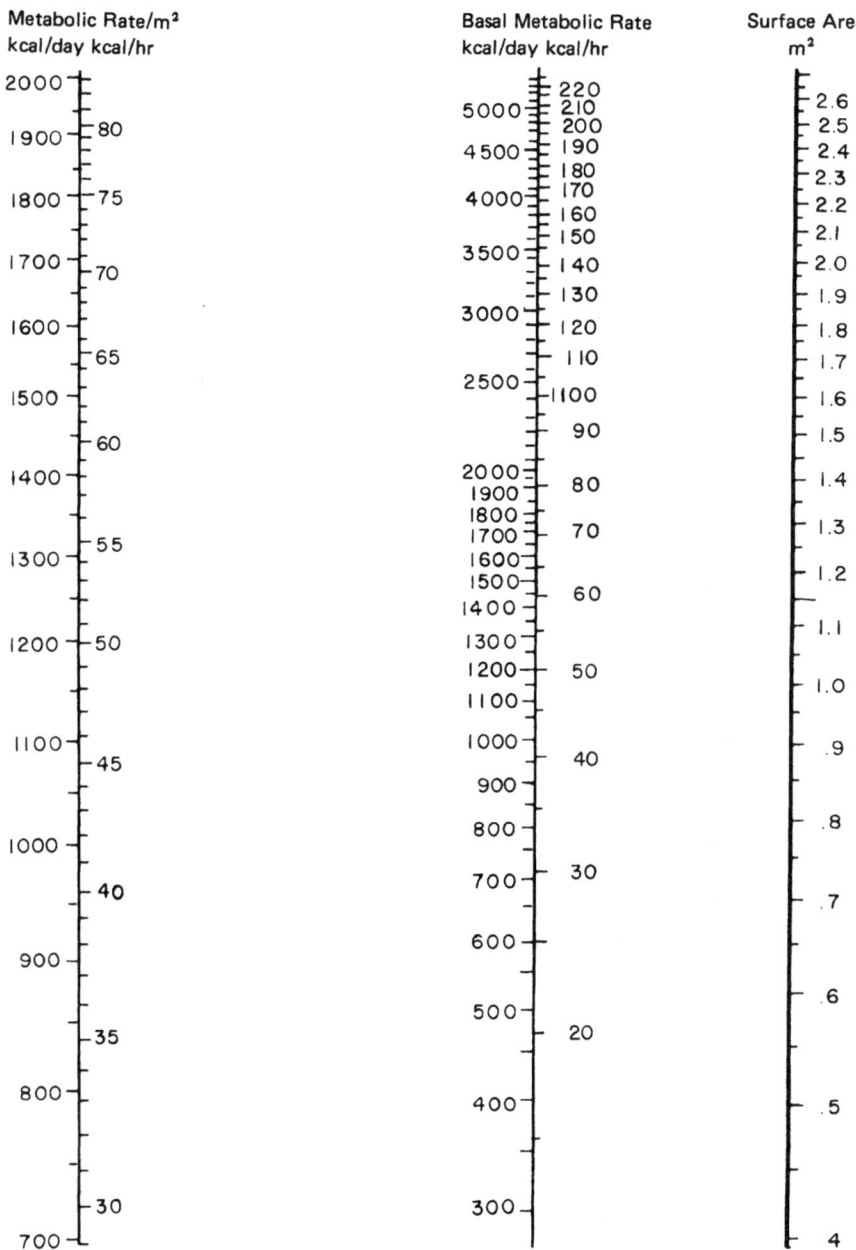

FIGURE 1.7: To predict daily metabolic requirements, determine surface area (right-hand scale) and metabolic requirements per m² body surface for age and sex (left-hand scale) (see Table 1.7). By connecting these points with a straightedge, the predicted daily or hourly requirements may be determined from the middle scale. To account for the impact of a disease process, remember the predicted daily metabolic rate and proceed to Fig. 1.11 (page 36).

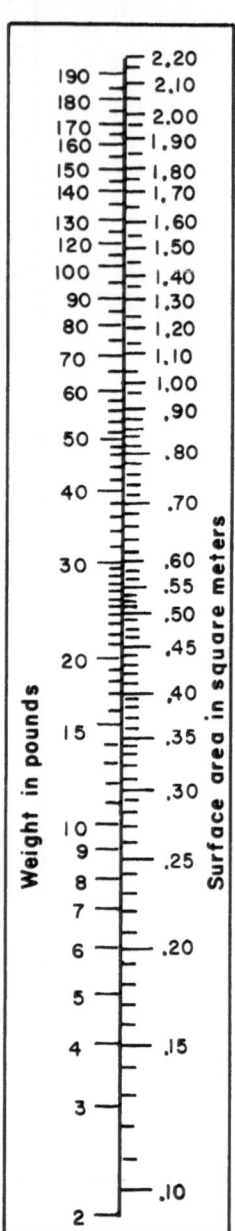

FIGURE 1.8: Body surface area of individuals of "normal" height may be read directly from the single scale.

Table 1.8   Metabolic Rate Calculated from Body Weight

Weight in lb	Weight in kg	Metabolic rate	
		kcal/hr ($3 \times wt^{0.75}$)	kcal/day ($70 \times wt^{0.75}$)
230.0	104.3	97.9	2285
229.3	104.0	97.7	2280
225.0	102.0	96.3	2247
224.9	102.0	96.3	2247
220.5	100.0	94.9	2214
220.0	99.8	94.7	2210
216.1	98.0	93.4	2180
215.0	97.5	93.1	2172
211.7	96.0	92.0	2147
210.0	95.2	91.5	2134
207.3	94.0	90.6	2113
205.0	93.0	89.8	2096
202.9	92.0	89.1	2079
200.0	90.7	88.2	2057
198.4	90.0	87.7	2045
195.0	88.4	86.5	2019
194.0	88.0	86.2	2011
190.0	86.2	84.8	1980
189.6	86.0	84.7	1977
185.2	84.0	83.2	1942
185.0	83.9	83.2	1941
180.8	82.0	81.7	1907
180.0	81.6	81.5	1901
176.4	80.0	80.2	1872
175.0	79.4	79.8	1861
172.0	78.0	78.7	1837
170.0	77.1	78.1	1821
167.6	76.0	77.2	1802
165.0	74.8	76.3	1781
163.2	74.0	75.7	1766
160.0	72.6	74.6	1740
158.8	72.0	74.2	1730
155.0	70.3	72.8	1699
154.3	70.0	72.6	1694
150.0	68.0	71.1	1658
149.9	68.0	71.0	1658
145.5	66.0	69.5	1621
145.0	65.8	69.3	1616
141.1	64.0	67.9	1584
140.0	63.5	67.5	1574

Continued

Table 1.8 — continued

		Metabolic rate	
Weight in lb	Weight in kg	kcal/hr ($3 \times wt^{0.75}$)	kcal/day ($70 \times wt^{0.75}$)
136.7	62.0	66.3	1547
135.0	61.2	65.7	1532
132.3	60.0	64.7	1509
130.0	59.0	63.8	1489
127.9	58.0	63.1	1471
125.0	56.7	62.0	1446
123.5	56.0	61.4	1433
120.0	54.4	60.1	1403
119.1	54.0	59.8	1394
115.0	52.2	58.2	1359
114.7	52.0	58.1	1356
110.3	50.0	56.4	1316
110.0	49.9	56.3	1314
105.8	48.0	54.7	1277
105.0	47.6	54.4	1269
101.4	46.0	53.0	1236
100.0	45.4	52.4	1223
97.0	44.0	51.3	1196
95.0	43.1	50.4	1177
92.6	42.0	49.5	1155
90.0	40.8	48.4	1130
88.2	40.0	47.7	1113
85.0	38.5	46.4	1083
83.8	38.0	45.9	1071
80.0	36.3	44.3	1035
79.4	36.0	44.1	1029
75.0	34.0	42.3	986
75.0	34.0	42.2	986
70.6	32.0	40.4	942
70.0	31.7	40.1	936
66.2	30.0	38.5	897
65.0	29.5	38.0	886
61.7	28.0	36.5	852
60.0	27.2	35.7	834
57.3	26.0	34.5	806
55.0	24.9	33.5	781
52.9	24.0	32.5	759
50.0	22.7	31.2	727

determined by exchangeable potassium.[15] More recently, oxygen consumption has been related over a wide range of ages to protein synthesis for growth or maintenance of the lean body mass.[16]

1.16   HOW DOES METABOLIC RATE VARY WITH AGE?

Heat production per square meter body surface area per unit time decreases steadily as infants approach puberty, then energy expenditure gradually decreases as age increases. This decrease is approximately 1–2% per decade in adults (20–75 years of age),[17] and is accounted for in many of the standard formulas which predict normal metabolic rate. The linear relationships between the early and late fall of metabolic rate are calculated from the standard metabolic rate data of Fleisch and shown below (Table 1.9).

Table 1.9   The Prediction of Metabolic Rate for Males and Females at Various Ages

Group	Age	Mathematical expression	r^2
Males	1–19	$y = 52.96 - 0.77x$	0.9651
Males	20–75	$y = 37.50 - 0.079x$	0.9366
Females	1–19	$y = 53.35 - 1.01x$	0.9816
Females	20–75	$y = 37.50 - 0.079x$	0.9366
All subjects	1–19	$y = 53.09 - 0.88x$	0.9766
All subjects	20–75	$y = 38.65 - 0.082x$	0.9773

x = Age in years.
y = Metabolic rate (kcal/m^2/hr).

These equations suggest that metabolic rate at any age can be predicted for all patients in the following manner:

1. Assuming a metabolic rate at age 0 of 55 kcal/m^2/hr, then, for each year of age up to 19 years, subtract one kcal, or

$$\text{Metabolic rate in kcal/m}^2\text{/hr} = 55 - \text{age}$$

[15]Kinney, J. M., Lister, J., and Moore, F. D.: Relationship of energy expenditure to total exchangeable potassium. *Ann. N.Y. Acad. Sci., 110*:711, 1963.

[16]Young, V. R., Steffee, W. P., Pencharz, P. B., Winterer, J. C., and Scrimshaw, N. S.: Total human body protein synthesis in relation to protein requirements at various ages. *Nature, 253*:192, 1975.

[17]Keys, A., Taylor, H. L., and Grande, F.: Basal metabolism and age of adult man. *Metabolism, 22*:579, 1973.

2. For patients older than 20 years, assume 37 kcal/m^2/hr for the basal metabolic rate for 20-year-old individuals and subtract 1 kcal for each 10 years over 20 years in age, or

$$\text{Metabolic rate in kcal/m}^2/\text{hr} = 37 - \left(\frac{\text{age} - 20}{10}\right)$$

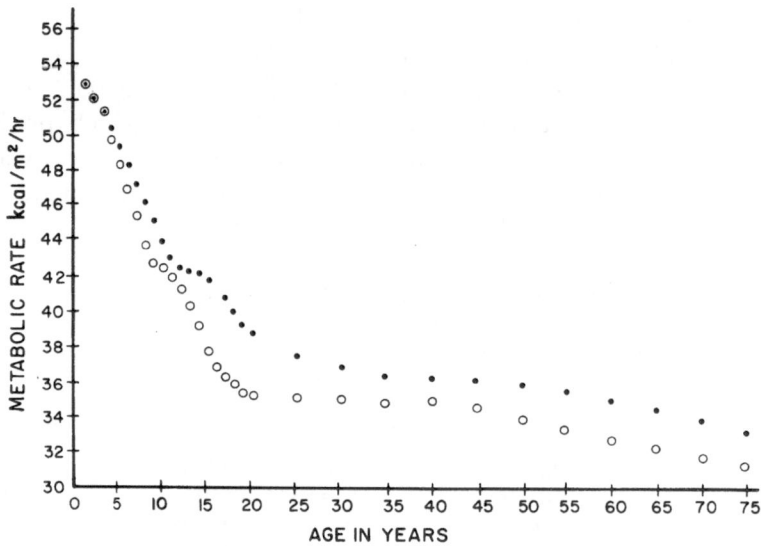

FIGURE 1.9: The effect of age on metabolic rate. (From the standards of Fleisch.) ● Men, ○ Women.

1.17   DOES THE SEX OF THE INDIVIDUAL AFFECT METABOLIC RATE?

Yes, a small sex difference exists in metabolic rate expressed per unit body surface area when comparing men and women. Females of comparable body size have slightly lower metabolic rates than men. This is accounted for in most predictive formulas or reference nomograms, and may be due to the slightly decreased lean body mass, or active metabolic tissue, and slightly increased fat mass which occurs in women of comparable surface area compared to men.

1.18   HOW DOES BODY TEMPERATURE AFFECT METABOLISM?

Metabolism and body temperature are dependent. As body temperature rises, there is an increase in the rate constant for chemical reactions, and, for each $10°C$, there is a two- to threefold increase in the reaction rate. This is known as the Q_{10} effect, and accounts for a 10–13% increase in heat production for each degree centrigrade rise in body temperature, although there is wide variation in this relationship in actual practice. Thus, the patient with a fever of $40°C$ may demonstrate an increase in oxygen consumption of 30–35% because of the elevation in body temperature alone. Conversely, hypothermia will decrease oxygen demands, and hypothermia is utilized in the operating room in patients who have interruption of the blood supply to vital organs (such as carotid reconstructive surgery in the elderly or cardiac surgery in infants) in order to decrease tissue oxygen demands and avoid tissue damage.

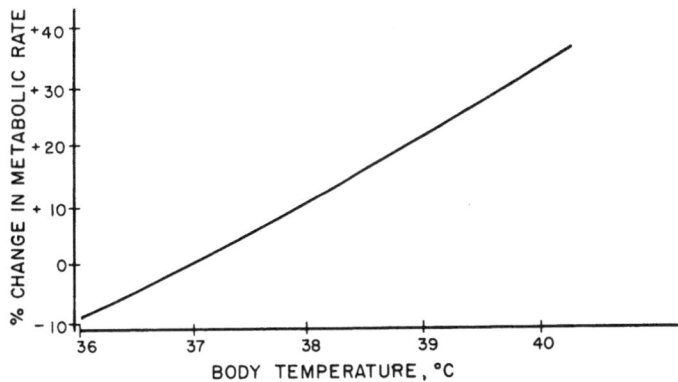

FIGURE 1.10: The effect of body temperature on metabolic rate. The coefficient for Q_{10} effect is calculated from an expected increase of 10% in oxygen consumption per $°C$. $M_T = 1.17633 \ (2.59374^{0.1t})$.

1.19   HOW DOES FOOD INTAKE AFFECT METABOLISM? WHAT IS SPECIFIC DYNAMIC ACTION?

Heat production of a subject under basal conditions increases above the basal level with food ingestion. This calorigenic effect of food is called "specific dynamic action" (often referred to as SDA, although the original description by Rubner[18] referred to "specific dynamic *effect*," not action). Protein exerts the greatest increase in heat production: if an individual is placed in a warm room, approximately 15% of the fed protein is dissipated as heat in the next 4 hr following ingestion of the foodstuff. This percentage is often quoted as high as 30% for protein, but, again, review of Rubner's data and examination of more recent research information suggest that the 30% calculation is too high. Studies in normals demonstrate that the specific dynamic effect for carbohydrate is 6% of ingested foodstuff, 2% for fat, 12% for protein-rich foods, but only 6% for a mixed diet. Others have accounted for a smaller quantity of energy production following food ingestion, particularly in febrile patients, critically ill individuals, and obese females.[19,20]

Initially, it was thought that the increased heat production following food ingestion was due to the energy cost of digestion. However, the injection of amino acid into the blood stream results in a comparable increase in heat production. In small animals, the increased oxygen consumption is confined to the viscera and not skeletal muscle following protein administration. No effect is observed if protein is injected into a hepatectomized animal. Krebs has accounted for the heat lost following protein ingestion as the energy cost of amino acid degradation and urea synthesis.[21] When the individual is exposed to a cold environment, the specific dynamic effect of food simply provides part of the heat required to maintain thermal balance, and heat produced following ingestion of food in a cold environment is not as pronounced as observed in a warm ambient temperature. Similarly, heat produced following protein ingestion is diminished in febrile, infected patients or hypermetabolic injured individuals.

Specific dynamic effect should be calculated as approximately 10% of the consumed calories when performing caloric balance

[18]Rubner, M.: *The Laws of Energy Consumption in Nutrition.* Leipzig and Vienna, Franz Deuticke, 1902.

[19]Bradfield, R. B., and Jourdan, M. H.: Relative importance of specific dynamic action in weight-reduction diets. *Lancet,* 2:640, 1973.

[20]Glickman, N., Mitchell, H. H., Lambert, E. H., and Keaton, R. W.: The total specific dynamic action of high-protein and high-carbohydrate diets in human subjects. *J. Nutr., 36*:41, 1948.

[21]Krebs, H.: The metabolic fate of amino acids. *In* Munro, H. N., and Allison, J. B., (Eds.): *Mammalian Protein Metabolism,* Vol. I. New York, Academic Press, 1964, p. 125.

calculations. Failure to account for this effect is a small error during exercise or in hypermetabolic, critically ill patients but produces a larger error in sedentary individuals.

1.20 HOW IS THE ENERGY EXPENDITURE OF ACTIVITY PREDICTED? HOW IS THE TOTAL DAILY ENERGY REQUIREMENT ESTIMATED?

Energy expenditure increases with muscular activity. This additional cost can be estimated by adding a caloric allowance for different grades of activity and work (see Table 1.10, p. 32). A more formal time—work study can be performed for precise determination of the total energy expenditures.[22]

   The total daily energy requirement is estimated in the following manner, where the numbers represent the estimated kcal/day for an active male white-collar worker:

1. Determine basal metabolism 1800
   (by measurement of oxygen consumption or from height—weight charts, adjusting for age and sex)
2. Estimate energy expenditure of activity 1000
   (use tables of hourly activity or application of time—work data)
3. Total basal + activity 2800
4. Add 10% for specific dynamic action of food 280

                                Total daily measurement   3080

1.21 WHAT IS THE EFFECT OF AMBIENT TEMPERATURE ON METABOLIC RATE?

Man controls heat loss and heat gain at thermal neutral temperatures by vasomotor regulation of skin blood flow and by altering sweat rate. Thus, dry and wet heat loss are controlled without major alterations in metabolic rate. As ambient temperature falls, a normal individual exposed to a cool environment responds by vasoconstriction to achieve core insulation and decreased sweat secretion.

[22]Consolazio, C. F., and Johnson, H. L.: Measurement of energy cost in humans. *Fed. Proc., 30*:1444, 1971.

Table 1.10   Approximation of Energy Costs
with Work

Type of work	Calories added to basal rates (kcal/day)
Sedentary	400–800
Light work (professionals and businessmen)	800–1200
Moderate work (mechanical)	1200–1800
Heavy work (laborers and athletes)[a]	1800–4500

[a]Caloric intakes of 9000 cal/day associated with maintenance of a stable body weight have been recorded in lumberjacks.

Further cooling results in hypermetabolism, which occurs in an individual with a normal or slightly decreased core temperature and a cool, dry skin. The central and peripheral temperature signals are integrated in the hypothalamus, and, when ambient temperature falls below 23–26°C, the sympathetic center of the central nervous system is stimulated and heat production above basal levels occurs. The ambient temperature at which the metabolic rate begins to rise above basal in order to maintain body temperature and heat balance is called the "critical temperature" (23–26°C in normal man).

Ambient temperatures above 37°C may exceed the ability of the body to lose the basal heat produced, primarily because secretion of sweat has achieved a maximal rate. As a result, core temperature rises and metabolic rate increases because of the increased tissue temperature (Q_{10} effect).

In most hospitalized patients, behavioral adaptation allows individuals to alter body insulation with blankets and bed clothing and thus maintain thermal neutrality or comfort. Responsive, oriented individuals will inform the hospital staff if they are too hot or too cold. In the critically ill patient, often unresponsive or sedated while receiving ventilatory support, behavioral adaptation to ambient temperature may not be possible. The stress of ambient temperature is an important effect in patients cared for in an air-conditioned intensive care area (a comfort level set for the pleasure of the staff and not the patients), with disease processes which cause alterations in temperature regulation (sepsis, head injury, thermal trauma, multiple injury). Patients placed in a cool, ambient temperature may be exposed to the additive stress of environmental temperature which may contribute to additional mortality and morbidity in selected patient groups.[23]

1.22   WHAT ALTERATIONS IN HEAT PRODUCTION OCCUR WITH STARVATION?

Heat production, and thus oxygen consumption, decreases with starvation. Heat production decreases to a greater degree than weight loss, and starved patients are hypometabolic if metabolic rate is expressed per unit body surface area. The decreased heat production which occurs in fasting man is probably related to the sudden fall in serum T_3 which occurs with fasting. Further alterations in heat production may be related to loss of active metabolic tissue from the body or may reflect a decrease in sympathetic activity associated with starvation. Decreased metabolic activity is manifest in partially or totally starved individuals by diminished muscle activity, increased sleep, fall in core temperature, and a constant requirement for external insulation to keep warm.

Table 1.11   Alterations in Basal Metabolic Rate Following a Prolonged Fast[a]

Day of fast:	1	21	31
kcal/day	1432	1002	1072
kcal/m²/day	904	664	737
kcal/kg/hr	1.07	0.87	0.99

[a]Subject Levanzin studied by Benedict.
Adapted from: Benedict, F. G.: *A Study of Prolonged Fasting*, Carnegie Institute of Washington, Publication No. 203, 1915.

1.23   TO WHAT EXTENT DOES INJURY OR INFECTION AFFECT ENERGY PRODUCTION?

Heat production increases with the size of injury or the extent of infection. As first described by Cuthbertson, long-bone fracture and

[23]Liljedahl, S. O., and Birke, G.: The nutrition of patients with extensive burns. *Nutr. Metab., 14* (Supp):110, 1972.

Table 1.12 The Best Estimates Available for Predicting Calorie Expenditure in Critically Ill Patients

Patient group	Author	Basal metabolic rate (range or ±SD of mean calculated value)
Normals	Dubois[a]	0 ± 12
Elective surgical		
Early (1−4 days)	Duke[b]	−1 ±16
Late (18−21 days)	Duke[b]	−4 ±16
Peritonitis	Duke[b]	+17 ±18
	Gump[c]	+17 ±15
Soft tissue trauma	Duke[b]	+14 ±17
Fracture	Cuthbertson[d]	+20 − +25
Infection (soft tissue, pneumonia, etc.)		
Mild	Dubois[a]	0 ± 20
Moderate	Dubois[a]	+20 − +40
Severe	Dubois[a]	+40 − +60
Typhoid fever	Coleman and Dubois[e]	+40 (occasional increases to +50)
Acute respiratory failure complicating sepsis	Halmagyi[f]	+60 ±18
Burn patients		
0−20%	Wilmore[g]	0 − +50
20−40%	Wilmore[g]	+50 − +85
40−100%	Wilmore[g]	+85 − +105
Burn injury with gram-negative bacteremia		
Mild	Wilmore[g]	10−20% below the value calculated for burn size
Severe	Wilmore[g]	20−60% reduction
Hyperthyroidism	Dubois[a]	+15 − +80
Hypothyroidism	Dubois[a]	−15 − −40
Malnutrition		
Children	Brooke[h]	−14
Adults	Keys[i]	−31

[a]Dubois, E.: *Basal Metabolism in Health and Disease.* New York, Lea and Febiger, 1924.

[b]Duke, J. H., Jorgensen, S. B., Broell, J. R., Long, C. L., and Kinney, J. M.: Contribution of protein to caloric expenditure following injury. *Surgery, 68:*168, 1970.

[c]Gump, F. E., Price, J. B., and Kinney, J. M.: Whole body and splanchnic blood flow and oxygen consumption measurements in patients with intraperitoneal infection. *Ann. Surg., 171:*321, 1970.

[d]Cuthbertson, D. P.: Observations on disturbance of metabolism produced by injury to the limbs. *Q. J. Med., 25:*233, 1932.

[e]Coleman, W., and Dubois, E.: Clinical calorimetry VII: Calorimetric observations on the metabolism of typhoid patients with and without food. *Arch. Int. Med., 15:*887, 1915.

[f]Halmagyi, D. F. J., and Kinney, J. M.: Metabolic rate in acute respiratory failure complicating sepsis. *Surgery, 77:*492, 1975.

[g]Wilmore, D. W., Long, J. M., Mason, A. D., Jr., Skreen, R. W., and Pruitt, B. A., Jr.: Catecholamines: Mediator of the hypermetabolic response to thermal injury. *Ann. Surg., 180:*653, 1974.

[h]Brooke, O. G., and Cocks, T. The metabolic rate of malnourished children. *J. Physiol. 231:*18p, 1973.

[i]Keys, A., Brožek, J., Henschel, A., Mickelsen, O., and Taylor, H. L.: *The Biology of Human Starvation,* Vol. 1. Minneapolis, University of Minnesota Press, 1950, p. 329.

soft-tissue injury produce a definite reproducible hypermetabolic state, with resting metabolic rates rising to 15–35% above normal. Kinney studied a variety of injured patients and found minimal changes in oxygen consumption following elective surgical procedures, but a gradual increase in metabolism with an increase in the extent of injury. Burn patients demonstrate the most prodigious increase in oxygen consumption, and patients with major thermal injury increase heat production at two times normal rates. It is rare, if ever, that metabolic demands exceed twice basal levels in the hospitalized patient studied supine in bed (Table 1.12).

1.24   WHAT IS THE ROLE OF PAIN, FEAR, AND ANXIETY IN HYPERMETABOLIC STATES?

The emotional response of a seriously ill individual may contribute to increased energy requirements of the disease process. Hume demonstrated that adrenal medullary response following cholecystectomy was greater in some patients who developed postoperative incisional pain, when compared with the stress of the operation itself.[24] Most of the measurements of oxygen consumption have been done in cooperative patients who are trained or acquainted with the use of respiratory equipment and are not anxious during the test conditions. Patients have been studied with tracheostomies, with or without ventilator support, and these tests confirm the fact that the increased oxygen consumption is not a form of anxiety. Patients have been studied with small doses of analgesics, and burn patients have been studied following deinnervation of their burn wound which rendered them free from pain. No alterations in the hypermetabolic response were observed. Thus, the disease process itself appears to stimulate the hypermetabolism. Pain, fear, and anxiety contribute to additional energy expenditure above the basal reset in metabolic rate. In some patients, analgesics and tranquilizers may be helpful in treating a component of the stress response. Every effort should be made to achieve patient comfort and minimize the additional stress which occurs as a result of a physician's therapy.

[24]Hume, D.: The endocrine and metabolic response to injury. *In* Schwartz, S. I. (Ed.): *Principles of Surgery*, New York, McGraw-Hill, 1969, p. 2.

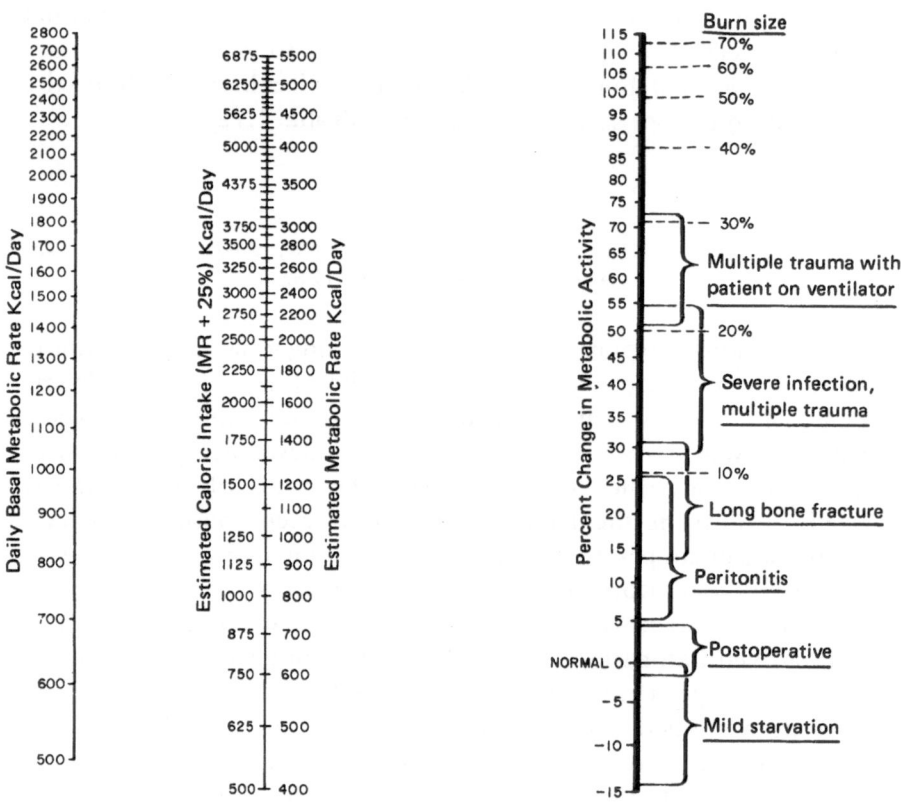

FIGURE 1.11: An estimate of energy requirements for critically ill patients.

1.25   HOW CAN THE ENERGY REQUIREMENT OF CRITICALLY ILL PATIENTS BE ESTIMATED?

1. Estimate the basal metabolic rate of the patient based on height, weight, age, and sex (Table 1.7, Fig. 1.7). This predicted value is an estimate of basal energy requirements when the individual is free of disease. Locate this value on the left-hand scale (Fig. 1.11).
2. Determine the impact of the disease state on basal metabolism by locating the disease on the right-hand scale.
3. By connecting the two points with a straightedge, the estimated metabolic rate is determined from the middle bar. Recommended caloric intake consists of estimated metabolic rate + 25%, and can be read from the left side of the middle bar.

1.26   WHAT IS ENERGY BALANCE?

Because man is an energy machine, the energy provided by the conversion of food into heat, work, growth, or fuel storage can be measured. When energy intake through food equals energy expenditure (Energy in = Energy out), a steady state is maintained and body weight remains constant. When food intake exceeds energy expenditure, the additional food is stored (primarily as fat), and the individual gains weight. When energy expenditure exceeds food intake, weight loss results. This relationship can be expressed as:

Energy balance (kcal/day) = Food intake (kcal/day)
                                    — Energy expenditure (kcal/day)

Positive energy balance is characteristic of weight gain and negative energy balance predictive of weight loss. The interactions between food intake and energy expenditure are best appreciated in the examples shown in Fig. 1.12.

1.27   HOW IS ENERGY BALANCE CALCULATED?

Each 3500 calories accounts for approximately one pound of body fat. While acute changes in body weight in critically ill patients

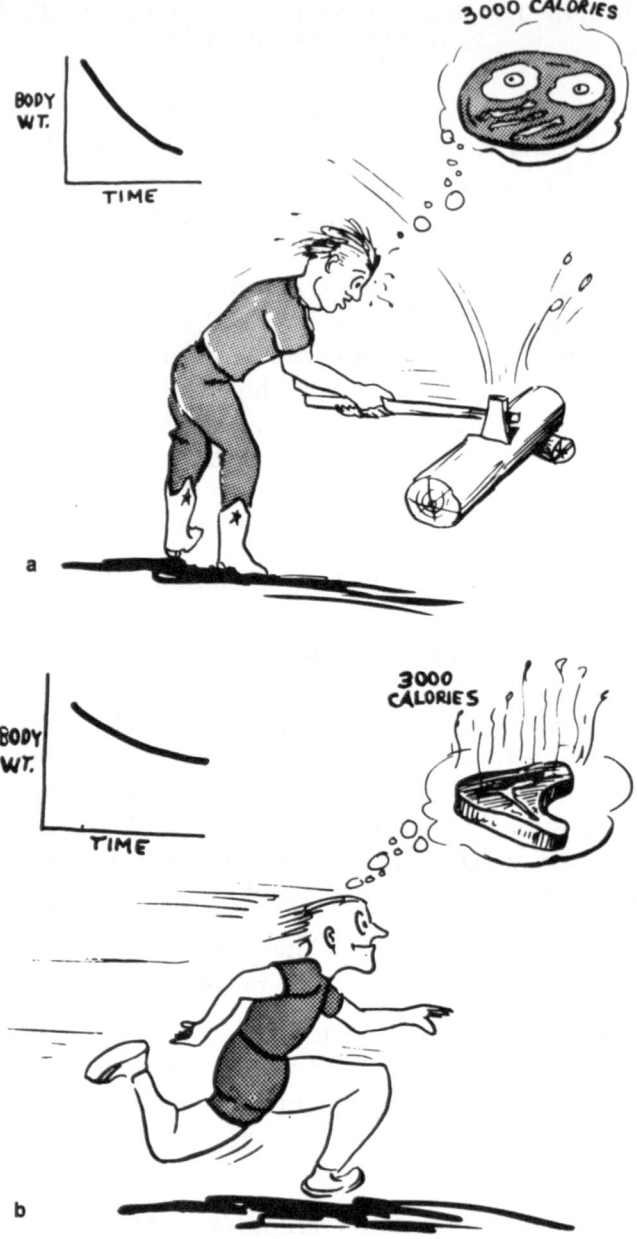

FIGURES 1.12a–d: Energy balance is a function of both food intake and energy expenditure. Note the alterations in body weight which occur with a constant food intake at four different activities.

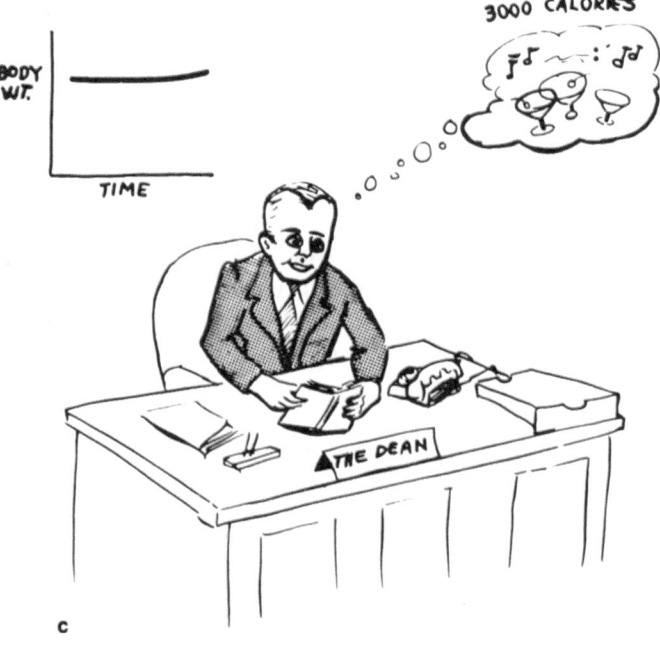

c

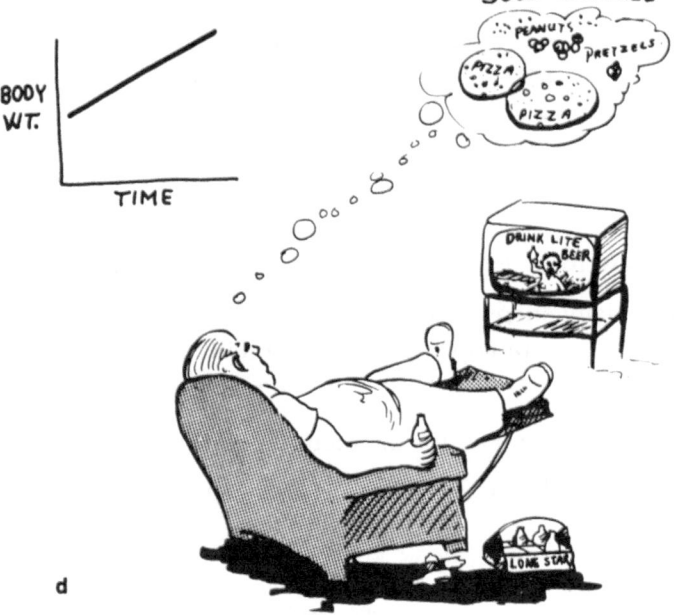

d

usually reflect alterations in total body water, long-term alterations in body weight reflect positive or negative energy balance. Kinney has emphasized that critically ill patients may gain up to 250 g of tissue per day, but that an increase in body weight in excess of this amount usually reflects positive fluid balance and not positive energy balance.[25]

Weight gain or weight loss can thus be calculated from the energy balance equation, although marked alterations in body weight result in a curvilinear relationship between body weight and time.[26] Weight loss not exceeding 10–15% of body mass may be calculated by this method with minimal error.

HOW MUCH WEIGHT LOSS WOULD OCCUR IN A 23-YEAR-OLD, SEDENTARY FEMALE, 5'3" TALL, WEIGHING 210 POUNDS, RECEIVING 1100 KILOCALORIES IN HER DIET EACH DAY FOR FOUR WEEKS?

1. Determine body surface area (Fig. 1.6, p. 21):

    5'3" female, 210 lb = 2 m^2 body surface area

2. Calculate basal energy expenditure (Table 1.7, p. 23):

    23-year-old female = 35 kcal/m^2/hr
    In 2 m^2 female   = 70 kcal/hr
    x 24 hr   = 1680 kcal/day

3. Estimate total daily caloric output (Table 1.10, p. 32):

Basal	=	1,680 kcal/day
Increase for sedentary activity	=	600 kcal/day
Total daily energy expenditure	=	2,280 kcal/day
or approximately		16,000 kcal/week
	or	64,000 kcal over 4 weeks

4. Calculate food intake for the dietary period:

    1100 kcal/day or 7700 kcal/week or 30,800 kcal/4 weeks

[25]Kinney, J. M., Long, C. L., Gump, F. E., and Duke, J. H., Jr.: Tissue composition of weight loss in surgical patients. I. Elective operations. *Ann. Surg.*, *168*:459, 1968.
[26]Antonetti, V. W.: The equations governing weight change in human beings. *Amer. J. Clin. Nutr.*, *26*:64, 1973.

5. Determine weight loss by the energy balance equation:

Calories in − Calories out = Calorie balance

30,800 kcal (in 4 weeks) − 64,000 kcal (burned in 4 weeks) =
−33,200 kcal (the caloric balance).

This deficit represents approximately 10 lb loss of body weight in 4 weeks (−33,200/3500 kcal/lb), or a loss in body weight of about 2.5 lb/week.

HOW MANY CALORIES SHOULD BE FED DAILY TO A 20-YEAR-OLD MALE, 5'8" TALL, WEIGHING 130 POUNDS, WITH A 70% BURN, TO PREVENT WEIGHT LOSS?

1. Determine body surface area: 1.7 m^2
2. Determine basal energy expenditure: 38.6 kcal/m^2/hr or 65.6 kcal/hr, or 1575 kcal/day
3. Estimate total daily caloric output (Fig. 1.11, p. 36): patients with large thermal injury increase metabolic rate approximately twice normal levels.

Daily caloric intake = 1575 x 2 = 3150 kcal/day

4. Determine caloric balance: since this patient should be maintained in caloric balance, then the energy intake equals the energy expenditure, that is, this man must receive a minimum of 3200 kcal/day throughout his hospitalization in order to prevent weight loss. Moreover, because of the increased metabolic demands above basal, the specific dynamic effect of food, and the periods of operative procedures which preclude food intake, we would increase this estimate approximately 15−25% to ensure adequate food intake. He would then be receiving approximately 4000 kcal/day.

A 35-YEAR-OLD FEMALE IS ADMITTED TO THE HOSPITAL WITH MALNUTRITION AND WEIGHT LOSS FOLLOWING SUBTOTAL GASTRECTOMY. SHE IS 5'2" TALL AND WEIGHS 70 POUNDS. HOW MANY CALORIES DOES SHE REQUIRE TO GAIN TWO POUNDS PER WEEK?

1. Determine body surface area: 1.20 m^2
2. Determine basal metabolic requirements: 35 kcal/m^2/hr, or 42 kcal/hr, or 1008 kcal/day.

3. Estimate total daily energy expenditure (Table 1.10, p. 32). The patient is confined to bed, and her additional requirements are no more than 20% of her basal needs.

Basal (1008 kcal) + 20% Additional kcal (202) =
Total energy expenditure of 1210 kcal.

4. Calculate energy balance: since this patient is to gain 2 lb per week, we need to provide a caloric excess of 7000 cal/week (1 pound = 3500 cal), or a caloric excess of 1000 kcal/day. Thus:

Food intake — Energy expenditure = +1000 kcal/day

or

Food intake = +1000 kcal/day + 1210 kcal/day
(daily energy expenditure)

or

Food intake = 2210 kcal/day

Add an additional 10% for the specific dynamic action of food:

Food intake + 10% = 2210 + 221 = 2431 kcal/day.

Food intake should be 2431 kcal/day to achieve weight gain of 2 lb/week.

1.28   HOW CAN THE WEIGHT ALTERATIONS OF PATIENTS BE PREDICTED?

Predict weight alterations from energy expenditure and food intake.

1. Estimate daily energy expenditure. Locate the point on the left-hand scale (Fig. 1.13).
2. Calculate food intake from an accurate calorie count. Locate point on right-hand scale marked energy intake.
3. By connecting the two parts, the weight loss over a week on this diet will be predicted on the middle scale.

Determine the number of calories for predicted weight gain or weight loss.

1. Determine energy expenditure. Locate point on left-hand scale.

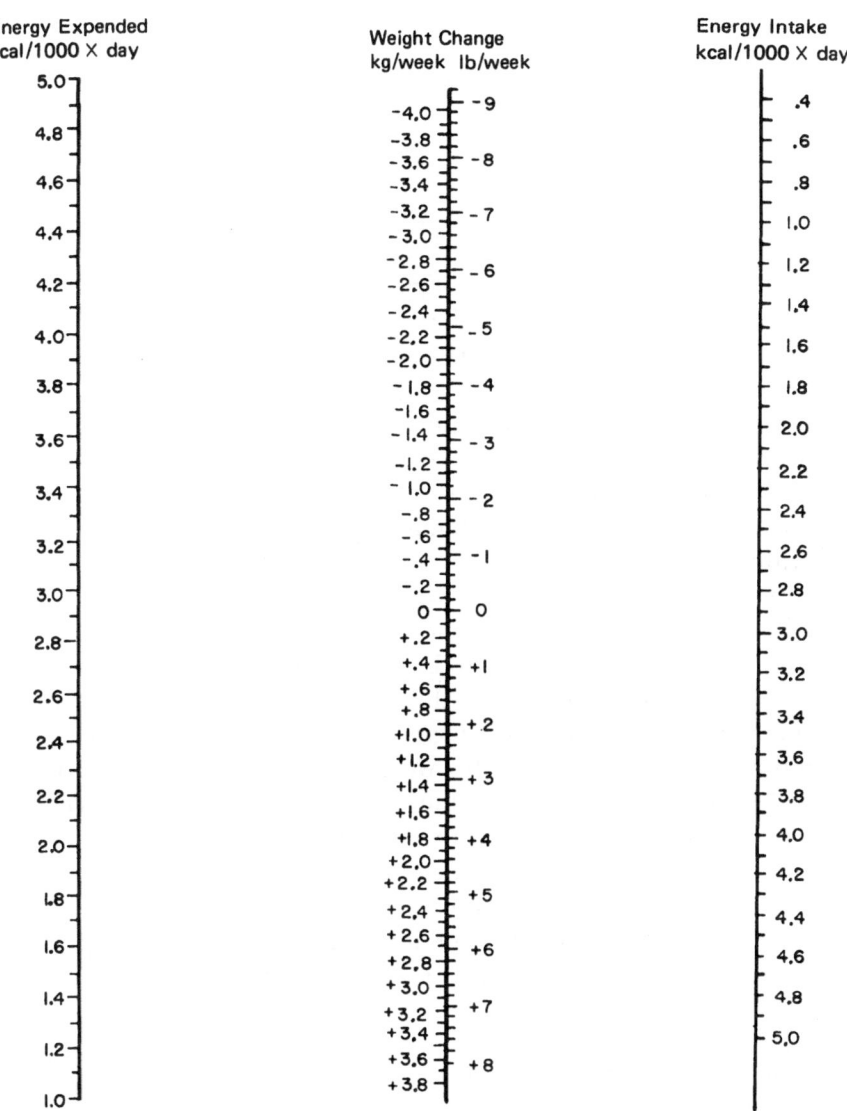

FIGURES 1.13: Predictions of weight alterations from estimated energy expenditure and food intake.

2. Locate desired weight gain or weight loss over a week on the middle scale.
3. By connecting the two points, the daily caloric value of the diet is determined on the right-hand scale to achieve this alteration in body weight.

1.29   TO WHAT EXTENT IS WEIGHT LOSS DETRIMENTAL?

Most data suggest that body-weight loss in excess of 10% normal body mass, associated with underhydration, results in rapid deterioration of maximal work performance.[27] Subjects evaluated in semistarvation studies for 10 days with weight loss less than 10% demonstrate no impairment in physical performance.[28] In addition, some authors suggest that altered physical performance is affected more by the rate of weight loss than the absolute extent of weight loss. The evidence from starvation in normal man (previously healthy individuals with normal body composition) suggests that a gradual weight loss of up to 10% body weight does not deleteriously affect physiologic function. The effect of weight loss in this range on immunological function is yet to be determined.

Loss of one-fourth to one-third protein mass from the body is predictably fatal,[29] and this degree of negative nitrogen balance in man is associated with a 40–50% weight loss. At some point between 10 and 40% body weight loss, malnutrition contributes to the disability of the previously healthy patient who had a normal body composition before injury.[30] Controlling the rate of weight loss and accepting more than 10% body weight loss only if resolution of a disease process can be assured in the immediate future are important guidelines for the nutritional care of critically ill individuals.

[27]Keys, A., Brožek, J., Henschel, A., Mickelsen, O., and Taylor, H. L.: *The Biology of Human Starvation*, Vol. 1. Minneapolis, Minn. University of Minnesota Press, 1950, pp. 714–746.

[28]Daws, T. A., Consolazio, C. F., Hilty, S. L., Johnson, H. L., Krzywicki, H. J., Nelson, R. A., and Witt, N. F.: Evaluation of cardiopulmonary function and work performance in man during caloric restriction. *J. Appl. Physiol., 33*:211, 1972.

[29]Montemurro, D. G., and Stevenson, J. A.: Survival and body composition of normal and hypothalamic obese rats in acute starvation. *Amer. J. Physiol., 198*:757, 1960.

[30]Studley, H. O.: Percentage of weight loss. A basic indicator of surgical risk in patients with chronic peptic ulcer. *J. Amer. Med. Assoc., 106*:458, 1936.

Table 1.13   Average Weights of Adults

Average weights in pounds and *kilograms* (in indoor clothing)

Height (in shoes)		15–16 years		17–19 years		20–24 years		25–29 years		30–39 years		40–49 years		50–59 years		60–69 years	
ft in	cm	lb	kg	lb	kg	lb	kg	lb	kg	lb	kg	lb	kg	lb	kg	lb	kg
											Men						
5 0	152.4	98	44.5	113	51.3	122	55.3	128	58.1	131	59.4	134	60.8	136	61.7	133	60.3
5 0½	153.7	100	45.4	114.5	51.9	123.5	56	129.5	58.7	132.5	60.1	135.5	61.5	137.5	62.4	134.5	61
5 1	154.9	102	46.3	116	52.6	125	56.7	131	59.4	134	60.8	137	62.1	139	63	136	61.7
5 1½	156.2	104.5	47.4	117.5	53.3	126.5	57.4	132.5	60.1	135.5	61.5	138.5	62.8	140.5	63.7	137.5	62.4
5 2	157.5	107	48.5	119	54	128	58.1	134	60.8	137	62.1	140	63.5	142	64.4	139	63
5 2½	158.8	109.5	49.7	121	54.9	130	59	136	61.7	139	63	142	64.4	143.5	65.1	140.5	63.7
5 3	160	112	50.8	123	55.8	132	59.9	138	62.6	141	64	144	65.3	145	65.8	142	64.4
5 3½	161.3	114.5	51.9	125	56.7	134	60.8	139.5	63.3	143	64.9	146	66.2	147	66.7	144	65.3
5 4	162.6	117	53.1	127	57.6	136	61.7	141	64	145	65.8	148	67.1	149	67.6	146	66.2
5 4½	163.8	119.5	54.2	129	58.5	137.5	62.4	142.5	64.6	147	66.7	150	68	151	68.5	148	67.1
5 5	165.1	122	55.3	131	59.4	139	63	144	65.3	149	67.6	152	68.9	153	69.4	150	68
5 5½	166.4	124.5	56.5	133	60.3	140.5	63.7	146	66.2	151	68.5	154	69.9	155	70.3	152	68.9
5 6	167.6	127	57.6	135	61.2	142	64.4	148	67.1	153	69.4	156	70.8	157	71.2	154	69.9
5 6½	168.9	129.5	58.7	137	62.1	143.5	65.1	149.5	67.8	155	70.3	158.5	71.9	159.5	72.3	156.5	71
5 7	170.2	132	59.9	139	63	145	65.8	151	68.5	157	71.2	161	73	162	73.5	159	72.1
5 7½	171.5	134.5	61	141	64	147	66.7	153	69.4	159	72.1	163	73.9	164	74.4	161	73
5 8	172.7	137	62.1	143	64.9	149	67.6	155	70.3	161	73	165	74.8	166	75.3	163	73.9
5 8½	174	139.5	63.3	145	65.8	151	68.5	157	71.2	163	73.9	167	75.8	168	76.2	165.5	75.1
5 9	175.3	142	64.4	147	66.7	153	69.4	159	72.1	165	74.8	169	76.7	170	77.1	168	76.2
5 9½	176.5	144	65.3	149	67.6	155	70.3	161	73	167.5	76	171.5	77.8	172.5	78.2	170.5	77.3
5 10	177.8	146	66.2	151	68.5	157	71.2	163	73.9	170	77.1	174	78.9	175	79.4	173	78.5
5 10½	179.1	148	67.1	153	69.4	159	72.1	165	74.8	172	78	176	79.8	177.5	80.5	175.5	79.6

Continued

Table 1.13—Continued

Average weights in pounds and *kilograms* (in indoor clothing)

Height (in shoes)		15–16 years		17–19 years		20–24 years		25–29 years		30–39 years		40–49 years		50–59 years		60–69 years	
ft in	cm	lb	kg	lb	kg	lb	kg	lb	kg	lb	kg	lb	kg	lb	kg	lb	kg
5 11	180.3	150	68	155	70.3	161	73	167	75.8	174	78.9	178	80.8	180	81.6	178	80.8
5 11½	181.6	152	68.9	157.5	71.4	163.5	74.2	169.5	76.9	176.5	80.1	180.5	81.9	182.5	82.8	180.5	81.9
6 0	182.9	154	69.9	160	72.6	166	75.3	172	78	179	81.2	183	83	185	83.9	183	83
6 0½	184.2	156.5	71	162	73.5	168	76.2	174.5	79.2	181	82.1	185	83.9	187	84.8	185.5	84.1
6 1	185.4	159	72.1	164	74.4	170	77.1	177	80.3	183	83	187	84.8	189	85.7	188	85.3
6 1½	186.7	161.5	73.3	166	75.3	172	78	179.5	81.4	185.5	84.1	189.5	86	191.5	86.9	190.5	86.4
6 2	188	164	74.4	168	76.2	174	78.9	182	82.6	188	85.3	192	87.1	194	88	193	87.5
6 2½	189.2	166.5	75.5	170	77.1	176	79.8	184	83.5	190.5	86.4	194.5	88.2	196.5	89.1	195.5	88.7
6 3	190.5	169	76.7	172	78	178	80.8	186	84.4	193	87.5	197	89.4	199	90.3	198	89.8
6 3½	191.8	—	—	174	78.9	179.5	81.4	188	85.3	196	88.9	200	90.7	202	91.6	201	91.2
6 4	193	—	—	176	79.8	181	82.1	190	86.2	199	90.3	203	92.1	205	93	204	92.5
Women																	
4 10	147.3	97	44	99	44.9	102	46.3	107	48.5	115	52.2	122	55.3	125	56.7	127	57.6
4 10½	148.6	98.5	44.7	100.5	45.6	103.5	46.9	108.5	49.2	116	52.6	123	55.8	126	57.2	128	58.1
4 11	149.9	100	45.4	102	46.3	105	47.6	110	49.9	117	53.1	124	56.2	127	57.6	129	58.5
4 11½	151.1	101.5	46	103.5	46.9	106.5	48.3	111.5	50.6	118.5	53.8	125.5	56.9	128.5	58.3	130	59
5 0	152.4	103	46.7	105	47.6	108	49	113	51.3	120	54.4	127	57.6	130	59	131	59.4
5 0½	153.7	105	47.6	107	48.5	110	49.9	114.5	51.9	121.5	55.1	128.5	58.3	131.5	59.6	132.5	60.1
5 1	154.9	107	48.5	109	49.4	112	50.8	116	52.6	123	55.8	130	59	133	60.3	134	60.8
5 1½	156.2	109	49.4	111	50.3	113.5	51.5	117.5	53.3	124.5	56.5	131.5	59.6	134.5	61	135.5	61.5
5 2	157.5	111	50.3	113	51.3	115	52.2	119	54	126	57.2	133	60.3	136	61.7	137	62.1

5 2½	158.8	112.5	51	114.5	51.9	116.5	52.8	120.5	54.7	127.5	57.8	134.5	61	138	62.6	139	63
5 3	160	114	51.7	116	52.6	118	53.5	122	55.3	129	58.5	136	61.7	140	63.5	141	64
5 3½	161.3	115.5	52.4	118	53.5	119.5	54.2	123.5	56	130.5	59.2	138	62.6	142	64.4	143	64.9
5 4	162.6	117	53.1	120	54.4	121	54.9	125	56.7	132	59.9	140	63.5	144	65.3	145	65.8
5 4½	163.8	119	54	122	55.3	123	55.8	127	57.6	133.5	60.6	141.5	64.2	146	66.2	147	66.7
5 5	165.1	121	54.9	124	56.2	125	56.7	129	58.5	135	61.2	143	64.9	148	67.1	149	67.6
5 5½	166.4	123	55.8	125.5	56.9	127	57.6	131	59.4	137	62.1	145	65.8	150	68	151	68.5
5 6	167.6	125	56.7	127	57.6	129	58.5	133	60.3	139	63	147	66.7	152	68.9	153	69.4
5 6½	168.9	126.5	57.4	128.5	58.3	130.5	59.2	134.5	61	140.5	63.7	149	67.6	154	69.9	155	70.3
5 7	170.2	128	58.1	130	59	132	59.9	136	61.7	142	64.4	151	68.5	156	70.8	157	71.2
5 7½	171.5	130	59	132	59.9	134	60.8	138	62.6	144	65.3	153	69.4	158	71.7	159	72.1
5 8	172.7	132	59.9	134	60.8	136	61.7	140	63.5	146	66.2	155	70.3	160	72.6	161	73
5 8½	174	134	60.8	136	61.7	138	62.6	142	64.4	148	67.1	157	71.2	162	73.5	163	73.9
5 9	175.3	136	61.7	138	62.6	140	63.5	144	65.3	150	68	159	72.1	164	74.4	165	74.8
5 9½	176.5	—	—	140	63.5	142	64.4	146	66.2	152	68.9	161.5	73.3	166.5	75.5	—	—
5 10	177.8	—	—	142	64.4	144	65.3	148	67.1	154	69.9	164	74.4	169	76.7	—	—
5 10½	179.1	—	—	144.5	65.5	146.5	66.5	150.5	68.3	156.5	71	166.5	75.5	171.5	77.8	—	—
5 11	180.3	—	—	147	66.7	149	67.6	153	69.4	159	72.1	169	76.7	174	78.9	—	—
5 11½	181.6	—	—	149.5	67.8	151.5	68.7	155.5	70.5	161.5	73.3	171.5	77.8	177	80.3	—	—
6 0	182.9	—	—	152	68.9	154	69.9	158	71.7	164	74.4	174	78.9	180	81.6	—	—

From K. Diem and C. Lentner (Eds.): *Scientific Tables*, 7th Ed., Ardsley, New York, Ciba-Geigy, 1971, p. 711.

Table 1.14   Desirable Weights of Adults

| Height (in shoes) | | Desirable weight in pounds and *kilograms* (in indoor clothing) for ages 25 and over | | | | | |
| | | Small frame | | Medium frame | | Large frame | |
ft in	*cm*	lb	*kg*	lb	*kg*	lb	*kg*
				Men			
5 2	*157.5*	112–120	*50.8–54.4*	118–129	*53.5–58.5*	126–141	*57.2–64*
5 3	*160*	115–123	*52.2–55.8*	121–133	*54.9–60.3*	129–144	*58.5–65.3*
5 4	*162.6*	118–126	*53.5–57.2*	124–136	*56.2–61.7*	132–148	*59.9–67.1*
5 5	*165.1*	121–129	*54.9–58.5*	127–139	*57.6–63*	135–152	*61.2–68.9*
5 6	*167.6*	124–133	*56.2–60.3*	130–143	*59 –64.9*	138–156	*62.6–70.8*
5 7	*170.2*	128–137	*58.1–62.1*	134–147	*60.8–66.7*	142–161	*64.4–73*
5 8	*172.7*	132–141	*59.9–64*	138–152	*62.6–68.9*	147–166	*66.7–75.3*
5 9	*175.3*	136–145	*61.7–65.8*	142–156	*64.4–70.8*	151–170	*68.5–77.1*
5 10	*177.8*	140–150	*63.5–68*	146–160	*66.2–72.6*	155–174	*70.3–78.9*
5 11	*180.3*	144–154	*65.3–69.9*	150–165	*68 –74.8*	159–179	*72.1–81.2*
6 0	*182.9*	148–158	*67.1–71.7*	154–170	*69.9–77.1*	164–184	*74.4–83.5*
6 1	*185.4*	152–162	*68.9–73.5*	158–175	*71.7–79.4*	168–189	*76.2–85.7*
6 2	*188*	156–167	*70.8–75.7*	162–180	*73.5–81.6*	173–194	*78.5–88*
6 3	*190.5*	160–171	*72.6–77.6*	167–185	*75.7–83.5*	178–199	*80.7–90.3*
6 4	*193*	164–175	*74.4–79.4*	172–190	*78.1–86.2*	182–204	*82.7–92.5*
				Women			
4 10	*147.3*	92–98	*41.7–44.5*	96–107	*43.5–48.5*	104–119	*47.2–54*
4 11	*149.9*	94–101	*42.6–45.8*	98–110	*44.5–49.9*	106–122	*48.1–55.3*
5 0	*152.4*	96–104	*43.5–47.2*	101–113	*45.8–51.3*	109–125	*49.4–56.7*
5 1	*154.9*	99–107	*44.9–48.5*	104–116	*47.2–52.6*	112–128	*50.8–58.1*
5 2	*157.5*	102–110	*46.3–49.9*	107–119	*48.5–54*	115–131	*52.2–59.4*
5 3	*160*	105–113	*47.6–51.3*	110–122	*49.9–55.3*	118–134	*53.5–60.8*
5 4	*162.6*	108–116	*49 –52.6*	113–126	*51.3–57.2*	121–138	*54.9–62.6*
5 5	*165.1*	111–119	*50.3–54*	116–130	*49 –59*	125–142	*56.7–64.4*
5 6	*167.6*	114–123	*51.7–55.8*	120–135	*54.4–61.2*	129–146	*58.5–66.2*
5 7	*170.2*	118–127	*53.5–57.6*	124–139	*56.2–63*	133–150	*60.3–68*
5 8	*172.7*	122–131	*55.3–59.4*	128–143	*58.1–64.9*	137–154	*62.1–69.9*
5 9	*175.3*	126–135	*57.2–61.2*	132–147	*59.9–66.7*	141–158	*64 –71.7*
5 10	*177.8*	130–140	*59 –63.5*	136–151	*61.7–68.5*	145–163	*65.8–73.9*
5 11	*180.3*	134–144	*60.8–65.3*	140–155	*63.5–70.3*	149–168	*67.6–76.2*
6 0	*182.9*	138–148	*62.6–67.1*	144–159	*65.3–72.1*	153–173	*69.4–78.5*

From: Weights of insured persons in the United States associated with lowest mortality. *Statist. Bull. Metrop. Life Insur. Co.*, 40, Nov.–Dec. 1959.

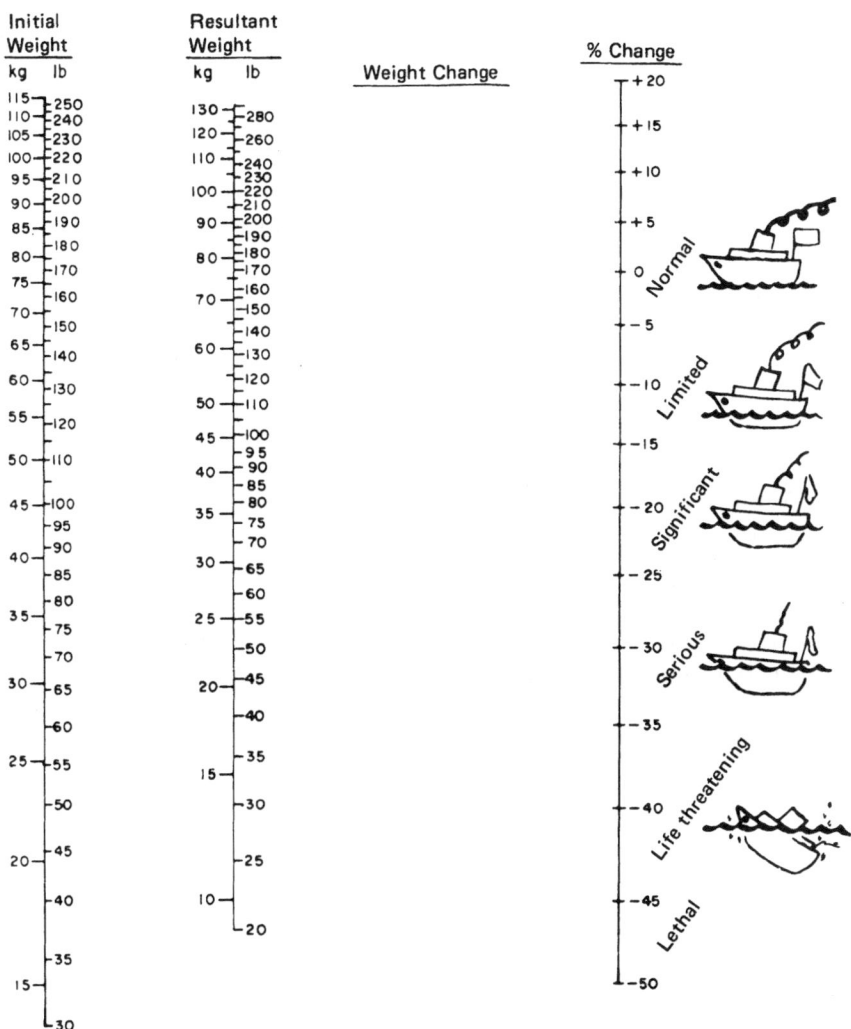

FIGURE 1.14: Alterations in nutritional status associated with weight loss.

However, patients with multiple injury, severe infection, or burns greater than 40% of body surface demonstrate a near-maximal stress response with predictable erosion of body mass. In these individuals, providing early protein and caloric support of at least predicted basal energy requirements is necessary for optimal care and may be essential for survival.

1.30   HOW IS THE NUTRITIONAL STATUS OF A PATIENT DETERMINED FROM BODY WEIGHT?

1. Have the patient give you his body weight *before* the onset of illness.
   (a) Is it normal? (Table 1.13, pp. 45–47)
   (b) Is it optimal? (Table 1.14, p. 48)
       Locate the weight on the left-hand scale (Fig. 1.14, p. 49).
2. Locate present weight on the middle of scale.
3. Connect the two points with a straightedge and read % change on right-hand scale.
   (a) Based on weight loss, what is the nutritional status of your patient?
   (b) Is more vigorous nutritional therapy indicated?
   (c) Is weight loss masked by retention of body fluid?

CHAPTER 2

Control of Body Temperature:
Relationships with Metabolic Control

2.1   WHY MEASURE ORAL OR RECTAL TEMPERATURE?

The mechanisms for control of body temperature are extremely efficient, but derangements in sensitivity of the central "thermostat" or alterations in the "setpoint" are frequently associated with disease. Elevation of body temperature is such a sensitive and reliable indication of the presence of a disease that thermometry is one of the most common and frequent measurements taken in hospitalized patients.

Core temperature (the temperature of deep or internal tissues) reflects the balance between heat production and heat loss from the body. Temperature may be elevated following strenuous exercise or after a hot bath. In contrast, a hypermetabolic patient may have a normal temperature if heat loss equals or exceeds the rate of heat production. In patients with fever secondary to infectious disease there is usually decreased heat loss from the body and increased heat storage. Metabolic rate is increased 10–13% with each 1°C rise in temperature, reflecting the Q_{10} temperature effect.

2.2   WHAT IS NORMAL BODY TEMPERATURE? WHAT ARE THE VARIATIONS IN BODY TEMPERATURE AROUND NORMAL?

Oral or rectal temperatures taken in a group of normal individuals demonstrate the usual bell-shaped distribution around a mean value.

Table 2.1   Conversion of Fahrenheit and Centigrade over the Range of Body Temperature [Conversion: $C = \frac{5}{9} (F - 32)$]

Fahrenheit	Centigrade	Fahrenheit	Centigrade	Fahrenheit	Centigrade
94.820	34.900	99.140	37.300	103.100	39.500
95.000	35.000	99.200	37.333	103.200	39.555
95.180	35.100	99.320	37.400	103.280	39.600
95.200	35.111	99.400	37.444	103.400	39.667
95.360	35.200	99.500	37.500	103.460	39.700
95.400	35.222	99.600	37.556	103.600	39.778
95.540	35.300	99.680	37.600	103.640	39.800
95.600	35.333	99.800	37.667	103.800	39.889
95.720	35.400	99.860	37.700	103.820	39.900
95.800	35.444	100.000	37.778	104.000	40.000
95.900	35.500	100.040	37.800	104.180	40.100
96.000	35.556	100.200	37.889	104.200	40.111
96.080	35.600	100.220	37.900	104.360	40.200
96.200	35.667	100.400	38.000	104.400	40.222
96.260	35.700	100.580	38.100	104.540	40.300
96.400	35.778	100.600	38.111	104.600	40.333
96.440	35.800	100.760	38.200	104.720	40.400
96.600	35.889	100.800	38.222	104.800	40.444
96.620	35.900	100.940	38.300	104.900	40.500
96.800	36.000	101.000	38.333	105.000	40.555
96.980	36.100	101.120	38.400	105.080	40.600
97.000	36.111	101.200	38.444	105.200	40.667
97.160	36.200	101.300	38.500	105.260	40.700
97.200	36.222	101.400	38.556	105.400	40.778
97.340	36.300	101.480	38.600	105.440	40.800
97.400	36.333	101.600	38.667	105.600	40.889
97.520	36.400	101.660	38.700	105.620	40.900
97.600	36.444	101.800	38.778	105.800	41.000
97.700	36.500	101.840	38.800	105.980	41.100
97.800	36.556	102.000	38.889	106.000	41.111
97.880	36.600	102.020	38.900	106.160	41.200
98.000	36.667	102.200	39.000		
98.060	36.700	102.380	39.100		
98.200	36.778	102.400	39.111		
98.240	36.800	102.560	39.200		
98.400	36.889	102.600	39.222		
98.420	36.900	102.740	39.300		
98.600	37.000	102.800	39.333		
98.780	37.100	102.920	39.400		
98.800	37.111	103.000	39.444		
98.960	37.200				
99.000	37.222				

In a quiet person, an oral temperature above 37°C (98.6°F) is usually an indication of disease and a temperature above 37.2°C (99°F) in a person who has been moderately active may have a similar significance. Rectal temperature is usually 0.3–0.6°C (0.5–1.0°F) higher than the oral measurement.

All individuals demonstrate periodic variations or rhythms in body temperature, and daily temperature variation may be as great as 1°C in normals. The highest temperature is usually in the afternoon and the increase has been attributed to activity and food ingestion. Core temperature falls with sleep and the lowest temperatures are usually recorded in the early morning. The average core temperature gradually falls with age.

2.3   HOW IS CORE TEMPERATURE MEASURED?

Temperature measurements of the body may be taken orally, rectally, in the esophagus, on the tympanic membrane, or in the vascular system. Rectal temperatures (taken 5–10 cm above the anal sphincter) are the most practical and reliable method of monitoring core temperatures in critically ill patients. However, response of rectal temperature to alterations of body temperature is slow. The esophagus offers an ideal location for temperature monitoring, but is practical only in the operating room when the patient is asleep. Tympanic temperature measurements may be generally related to core temperature and are useful if ambient temperature is constant; alterations in tympanic membrane temperature may correlate with alterations in mean body temperature.[1]

Intravascular temperature measurements determine regional temperature variations and may be utilized to calculate organ heat production and regional heat flow. With the use of thermal dilution cardiac output catheters, a central intravascular thermistor is often available for continuous measurement of central intravascular temperature. Measurements in normal man demonstrate that rectal temperature is consistently 0.2–0.3°C above right-heart temperature while in the steady state. This difference increases in critically ill

---

[1] Nadel, E. R., and Horvath, S. M.: Comparison of tympanic membrane and deep body temperature in man. *Life Sci.,* 9:869, 1970.

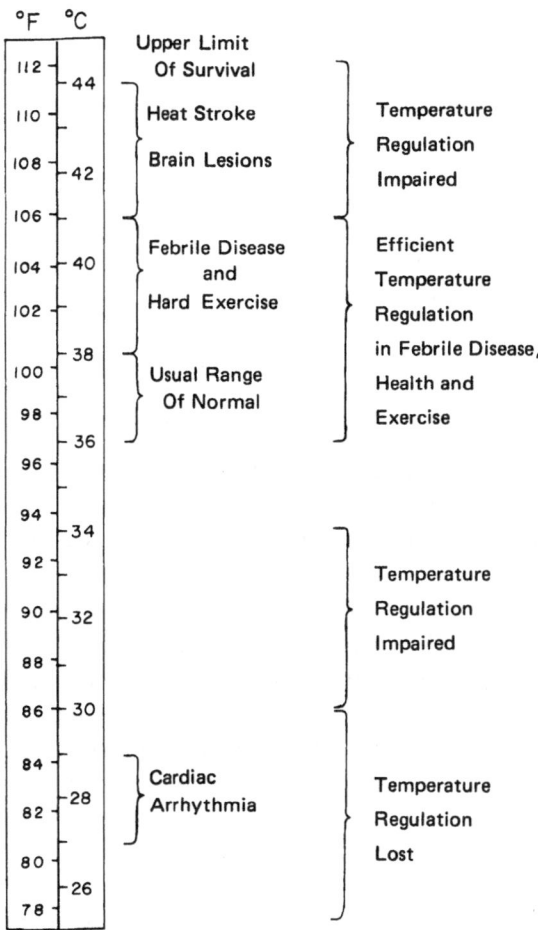

FIGURE 2.1: Variations and consequences of extreme body temperature (adapted from: DuBois, E. F.: *Fever and the Regulation of Body Temperature*, p. 9, Springfield, Ill., Charles C Thomas, 1948).

patients and rectal temperature may exceed intracardiac temperature by as much as 0.8°C during fever.[2]

2.4   HOW ARE MEAN SKIN TEMPERATURE AND MEAN BODY TEMPERATURE DETERMINED?

Mean skin temperature is a weighted calculation derived from multiple temperature measurements of the skin surface. Classically, 15 points have been measured and then mathematically weighted for surface area to determine mean skin temperature:

$$T_{skin} = 0.07 \times T_{feet} + 0.32 \times T_{legs} + 0.18 \times T_{chest} + 0.17 \times T_{back} + 0.14 \times T_{arms} + 0.05 \times T_{hands} + 0.07 \times T_{head}$$

Other investigators have utilized the mean or weighted mean of four to six specific skin points as a practical approach to determining mean skin temperature, measurements that may be applicable to experimental work under some circumstances.

Some clinicians have utilized measurements obtained from a single thermocouple placed on the finger or toe.[3] Marked changes in a single skin temperature reflect peripheral vasomotor alterations. The most important information from a single digital temperature measurement is the change or Δ temperature that occurs with time, which may correlate with alterations in core temperature observed during the same time period. Changes in the single digital temperature may not reflect generalized alterations in skin blood flow.

Mean body temperature is estimated from a weighted average of the core temperature (rectal, esophageal, or intravascular) and skin temperature. The usual weighting factors are:

$$T_{mean\ body} = 0.3 T_{skin} + 0.7 T_{rectum}$$

[2]Eichna, L. W., Berger, A. R., Rader, B., and Becker, W. H.: Comparison of intracardiac and intravascular temperatures with rectal temperatures in man. *J. Clin. Invest., 30*:353, 1951.

[3]Molnar, G. W., and Read, R. C.: An analysis of postoperative pyrexia. *J. Surg. Res., 17*:79, 1974.

The constants should be altered with marked changes in environmental temperature; in cold environments, the constant by which skin temperature is multiplied should be dropped to 0.2, and in warm environments raised to 0.4, with the constant for core temperature altered accordingly.

2.5   HOW IS HEAT LOST FROM THE BODY?

Heat is lost from the body by the wet and dry routes. Since in the steady state, heat lost from the body may be equated with heat gain, this relationship can be expressed in the following manner:[4]

Heat production = Heat of evaporation + Heat of radiation
+ Heat of conduction + Heat of convection

Table 2.2   Routes of Heat Loss

Mechanisms of heat loss	Route	Transfer	% Loss in average man/day
Wet	Evaporation	Skin to air	21
		Respiratory tree to air	4
Dry	Radiation	Skin to external radiating surfaces	44
	Conduction	Skin to contact surfaces	31
	Convection	Skin to air	

2.6   HOW IS EVAPORATIVE WATER LOSS MEASURED?

Wet heat loss occurs primarily with the vaporization of water; as water passes from a liquid to a gaseous state, thermal energy is required. The latent heat of vaporization of water is 580 kcal/liter, or 0.58 kcal/g of water vaporized. Evaporative water loss is usually

[4]Hardy, J. D.: Heat transfer. In L. H. Newburgh (Ed.): *Physiology of Heat Regulation and the Science of Clothing.* New York, Hofner, 1968, p. 78.

measured on a carefully calibrated bed scale.[5] After equilibrium has been reached by the patient with ambient temperature and humidity, serial body weights are taken (no loading or unloading of the scale is permitted during the measurement) and the rate of weight loss is determined. The water lost by the evaporative route is a combination of water lost from the skin and from the respiratory tree. Respiratory water loss is a function of the rate of pulmonary gas exchange, for even at high ventilatory rates, expired air is almost completely saturated with water. By measuring oxygen consumption, water loss from the respiratory tree can be estimated and the latent heat of vaporization due to respiration calculated.[6]

Heat lost by the insensible water route is relatively small and, in individuals resting in a thermal-neutral or cool environment, it accounts for 15—25% of the total heat lost. However, in warm environments or following generation of an internal heat load, sweat glands are stimulated and the quantity of water elaborated is directly proportional to the sweat gland stimulation, although decreased sweat secretion may accompany dehydration. The ability of water to remove heat from the body depends not only on the sweat rate but also on the ability of the environment to remove water vapor. Environmental factors which affect water loss from the surface include wind velocity over the surface and the partial pressure of water of the environmental air; the difference between the partial pressure of water on the surface and in the air is the driving force for water vapor movement.

2.7   HOW DOES FEVER AFFECT EVAPORATIVE WATER LOSS? WHAT OTHER DISEASES ALTER INSENSIBLE WATER LOSS?

Approximately 1 liter of water per day is lost by the insensible route in the typical patient. As previously noted, a variety of factors affect insensible water loss, including ambient temperature, partial pressure of water in the environment, wind velocity, and internal heat drive of the individual.

---

[5]Bradham, G. B., Thompson, N. J., and Reynolds, J. C.: The use of a metabolic scale. *J. Amer. Med. Assoc., 198*:746, 1966.

[6]Mitchell, J. W., Nadel, E. R., and Stolwijk, J. A. J.: Respiratory weight losses during exercise. *J. Appl. Physiol., 32*:474, 1972.

Many febrile, critically ill patients may lose up to 2 liters of water by the insensible route each day, and this is rarely accounted for solely by water loss from the respiratory tract.[7] However, most patients receiving humidified air or gas mixtures by face mask, or requiring ventilatory support by a mechanical respirator, inhale a totally saturated gas mixture. Under these conditions, respiratory water loss is minimal and positive water loading by way of the pulmonary tree may occur.

Adult patients who are small and hypometabolic (secondary to partial or total starvation) have measured rates of evaporative water loss of 500–600 ml/day. Rigid fluid restriction is necessary if gradual unloading of excessive body water by evaporation is expected.

Finally, patients who have a damaged or diseased integument, such as thermally injured patients, lose the water vapor pressure barrier of the skin and have large insensible water losses. In the burn patient, evaporative water loss is related to burn size and may be predicted by the nomogram shown in Fig. 2.2.

2.8   WHAT ARE THE ROUTES OF DRY HEAT LOSS?

The major portion of heat lost from the body is by the dry routes: radiation, convection, and conduction. The total dry heat loss may be calculated in the steady state by assuming:

$$\text{Heat production} = \text{Heat loss}$$

then

Heat production (determined by measurement of $\dot{V}_{O_2}$ and $\dot{V}_{CO_2}$) in $kcal/m^2/hr$ − Evaporative loss in $g/m^2/hr \times 0.58 \ kcal/g =$
$$\text{Dry heat loss in } kcal/m^2/hr$$

Dry heat loss may also be measured directly in a direct calorimeter.

Radiation is the major route of dry heat loss. The exchange of energy by radiation depends upon the temperature of the surfaces which radiate to each other and the radiating quality of these surfaces. Radiative heat loss does not depend upon the temperature

[7]Roe, C. F., and Kinney, J. M.: Water and heat exchange in third-degree burns. *Surgery*, *56*:212, 1964.

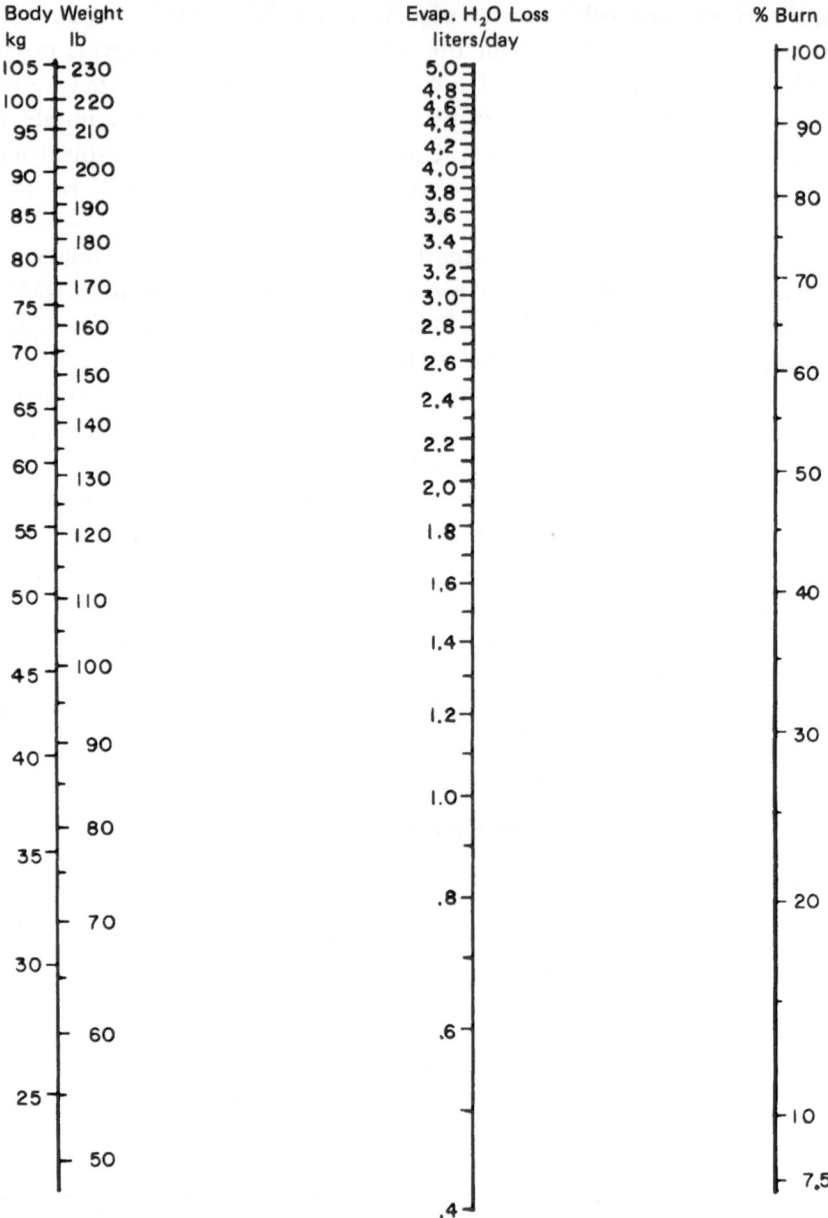

FIGURE 2.2: Prediction of water loss in thermally injured patients based on body weight and percent body surface area burn.

of the air between the surfaces. Radiative heat loss may be calculated from the Stefan—Boltzmann equation:

$$H_r \text{ (kcal/hr)} = 1.37 \times 10^{-11} (T_s^4 - T_c^4) \times t \times A \times f \times e$$

where T_s is the average skin temperature ($^\circ$C + 273), T_c is the average radiative environmental temperature (wall temperature in $^\circ$C + 273), t is the number of seconds in an hour, A is the body surface area, f is the ratio of effective radiating surface (0.5 for men supine in bed), and e is the emissivity of the environment (0.95 for white lacquered walls).

Heat loss by convection depends on the movement and density of the environmental medium, whether air or water. Convective heat loss depends upon the temperature gradient between the body surface and the ambient air, the exposed body surface area, and the velocity of air flow over the surface. The chill we perceive when sitting in a draft is due to increased convection. The increased heat

Table 2.3   Heat Loss in Normals and Patients with Altered Evaporative Water Loss Studied at 25 and 33°C Ambient Temperature

Ambient temperature ($^\circ$C)	Normals ($n = 4$)		Anhydrotic ectodermal dysplasia[a] ($n = 2$)		Burns ($n = 8$)	
	25	33	25	33	25	33
Metabolic rate (kcal/m^2/hr)	35.6	36.3	39.1	38.0	63.5	62.0
Evaporative water loss (g/hr)[b]	28.7	93.4	8.7	14.5	94.3	148.7
% of heat lost						
Evaporation	22.7	73.8	7.1	15.5	44.8	73.6
Radiation	46.0	8.8	90.1	38.3	33.0	14.0
Conduction and convection	31.3	17.4	2.8	46.2	22.2	12.4

[a]Congenital absence of sweat glands.

[b]Note the increase in wet heat loss in normals which occurs with an elevation in ambient temperature. Patients unable to lose heat by evaporation are similar to normals in the cooler environment while burn patients with increased evaporative water loss have a similar proportion of wet and dry heat loss when compared to normals in the warmer environment.

Adapted from: Wilmore, D. W., Mason, A. D., Jr., Johnson, D. W., and Pruitt, B. A., Jr.: Effect of ambient temperature on heat production and heat loss in burn patients. *J. Appl. Physiol.*, *38*:593, 1975.

loss which is accounted for during the chill phase of an infection may be due to increased air movement at the body surface, created by the vibrations and shivering of the chill which stirs the air around the body.

The heat loss by conduction concerns only that part of the body in contact with other materials. This is of little importance in a standing man, but plays a more important role in patients lying supine on a mattress. Water-impermeable mattress covers are good insulators and the skin temperature of the back in most supine patients approaches rectal temperature.

2.9   HOW DOES MAN INSULATE BETWEEN HIS SKIN AND THE SURROUNDING ENVIRONMENT?

Most of man's adaptations to alterations in environmental temperature are determined by behavioral changes: he alters his body posture to minimize surface area exposure or adds clothing to provide greater body insulation. Most hospitalized patients utilize bed clothing and covers to provide adequate skin—air insulation. In patients with open wounds, a bed cradle covered with blankets will cocoon the individual and provide a microenvironment that may provide a satisfactory comfort temperature for the patient. Room temperature may be regulated to satisfy patient comfort or heat lamps may be placed around the individual to provide additional radiant heat.

Calculations for heat loss from the body to the environment are based on some estimate of the exposed portion of the body surface area. In a man standing upright with his legs together and his arms close to his side, about 80% of the body surface area is involved in effective heat exchange. Patients in bed have their backs overcoated by the mattress and the exposed area is reduced to approximately 50—60%. If a man assumes the fetal position by curling up, the exposed surface area for heat exchange is reduced even more while a supine man in the spread-eagle position maximizes the surface area exposed while in bed.

2.10   WHAT DETERMINES HEAT FLOW TO THE BODY SURFACE? WHAT IS CONDUCTANCE?

Gradients exist between the areas of central heat production and the skin surface. Heat may move to the surface for dissipation by conduction through the tissues, but all body tissues are poor conductors and hence little heat exchange occurs solely by this method.

The movement of heat from the central core — at rest most heat is generated by the brain and visceral tissue — to the peripheral tissues is effected by the circulatory system. The rich circulation in the skin and subcutaneous tissue carries heat from the deeper portions of the body to the surface where it can escape. Once heat is moved to the surface, it can be dissipated from the skin by wet or dry routes of heat transfer. When there is a requirement for increased heat transfer to the periphery, vasodilatation occurs. Skin temperature may increase but, if sweating occurs, the surface will be cooled by evaporation and surface temperature may not change, or may actually decrease. Conversely, body heat conservation occurs with vasoconstriction. Heat is also conserved in the extremities by countercurrent exchange mechanisms. Decreased circulation to the surface alters the insulative layer around the body, minimizing body heat loss, and facilitating body heat storage.

Conductance or core—skin heat transfer is a measure of heat flow from the central core to the surface. Conductance is calculated from metabolic rate, core temperature, and skin temperature:

$$\text{Conductance in kcal/m}^2/{}^\circ\text{C/hr} = \frac{\text{Metabolic rate kcal/m}^2/\text{hr}}{T_{core} - T_{skin}}$$

Conductance varies inversely with insulation, and is reduced to a minimum during cold exposure (Fig. 2.3). The inability to reduce skin blood flow during sepsis, burn trauma, and some forms of peripheral vascular disease has been measured by this technique (Table 2.4): peripheral blood flow may also be calculated from these measurements or measured directly.

2.11   WHAT ALTERATIONS IN CORE–SKIN HEAT TRANSFER ARE OBSERVED IN PATIENTS?

Obese patients have a greater insulative layer because of their increased fat mass, which reduces core—skin heat transfer during cold exposure.[8] Patients with congestive heart failure fail to dilate the cutaneous circulation in response to a thermal stress because of

[8]Jequier, E., Gygax, P.-H., Pittet, P., and Vannotti, A.: Increased thermal body insulation: Relationship to the development of obesity. *J. Appl. Physiol.*, *36*:674, 1974.

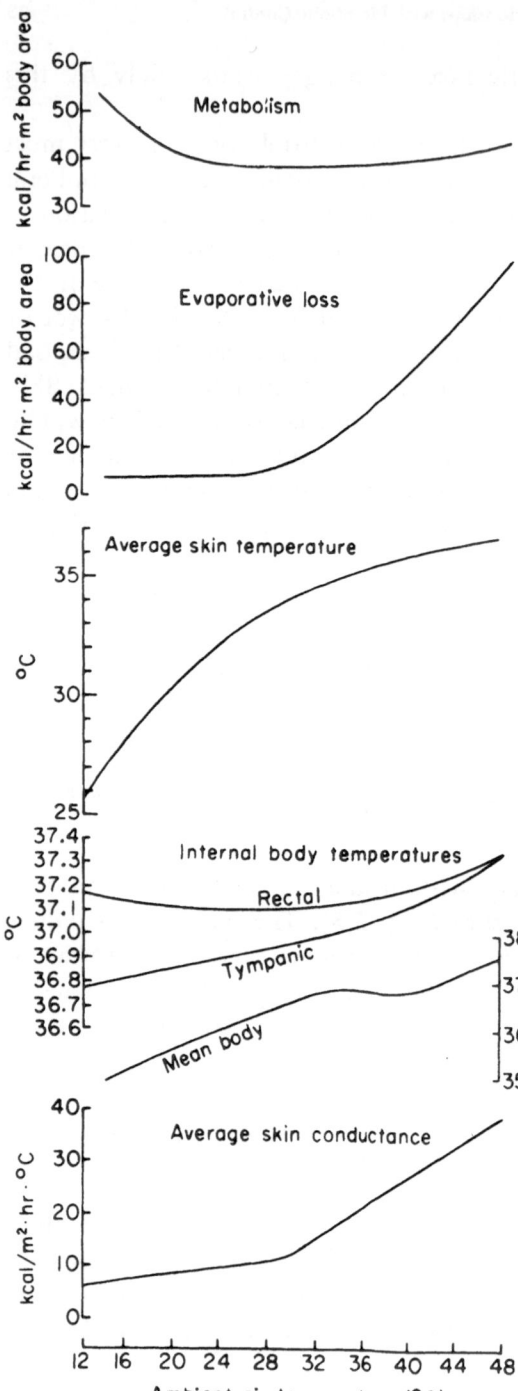

FIGURE 2.3: Alterations in metabolism, evaporative loss, body temperature, and conductance with alterations in ambient temperature (adapted from Hardy, J. D., Stolwijk, J. A. J., and Gagge, A. P. *In*: G. C. Whittow (Ed.): *Comparative Physiology in Thermoregulation*, Vol. 2. New York, Academic Press, 1971, p. 336.

Table 2.4   Alterations in Conductance and Heat Transfer Coefficients in
Normals and Patients with Altered Evaporative Water Loss[a]

	Normals		Anhydrotic ectodermal dysplasia		Burns	
Ambient temperature ($^\circ$C)	25	33	25	33	25	33
Core temperature ($^\circ$C)	36.8	36.8	37.1	38.0	38.5	38.0
Mean skin temperature ($^\circ$C)	31.4	34.2	33.2	36.3	33.1	36.2
Core-to-skin (kcal/m^2/hr/$^\circ$C; conductance)	6.64	14.21	10.22	22.56	12.70	26.32
Core-to-air (kcal/m^2/hr/$^\circ$C)	3.01	9.62	3.23	7.46	4.73	11.28
Core-to-air (dry) (kcal/m^2/hr/$^\circ$C)	2.33	2.51	3.10	6.56	2.56	2.74

[a]Note the variations in skin temperature and core-to-skin heat transfer coefficient (conductance) which occur between patient groups and with alterations in ambient temperature (conductance moves inversely with insulation). Patients without mechanisms for sweating have maximum vasodilatation to warm the skin and establish increased heat loss by the dry routes. In the patients studied, this mechanism was inadequate for dissipation of body heat in the 33°C ambient temperature and core temperature rose to 38°C. Burn patients have increased conductance at any ambient temperature studied, because increased blood flow to the wound occurs.

increased sympathetic alpha adrenergic tone and increased circulating catecholamines. These individuals cannot transport increased internal heat to the surface in a normal manner and frequently demonstrate slight temperature elevations, especially following mild exertion.[9]

Septic patients and individuals with thermal injury and extensive exfoliative skin disease have increased skin blood flow and cannot adequately reduce blood flow and insulate when exposed to a cold environment. This explains in part the hypothermia which may occur in these patients, especially when exposed to a cool ambient temperature.

2.12   HOW DOES THE BRAIN CONTROL BODY TEMPERATURE?

Man is a homotherm, able to maintain body temperature within narrow limits. The regulation of body temperature occurs principally through the dynamic action of the autonomic nervous system which

[9]Zelis, R., Nellis, S. H., Longhurst, H., Lee, G., and Mason, D. T.: Abnormalities in the regional circulation accompanying congestive heart failure. *Prog. Cardiovas. Dis.*, *18*:181, 1975.

regulates vasomotor tone, stimulates or inhibits exocrine or endo-crine glands, and simultaneously alters metabolic rate, substrate flow, and respiratory rate. An intact brain stem is essential for body temperature regulation, and appropriate autonomic adjustment occurs in response to external temperature change of even the slightest magnitude. In 1885 Aronsohn and Sachs described the presence of a temperature regulating center in the anterior hypo-thalamus which protects against overheating in a warm environment (heat dissipation center). Animals with lesions in this portion of the hypothalamus can regulate body temperature when placed in a cold environment but overheat in a warm environment. A second area of temperature regulation is located in the posterior hypothalamus, and is indispensable for chemical regulation of heat production in cold environments (heat conservation center). This area lies within the sympathetic area of the hypothalamus, and animals with lesions in this center fail to vasoconstrict and shiver when exposed to a cold environment, although they thermally regulate appropriately when exposed to warm environments. The thermal regulatory areas are closely integrated in their responses; some authors feel that the anterior center is dominant and controls both heat dissipation and heat conservation. The thermoregulatory areas are similarly located in humans and severe hyperthermia and hypothermia have been associated with hypothalamic lesions in man.

2.13   WHAT IS TEMPERATURE SETPOINT? WHAT FACTORS ALTER SETPOINT?

The temperature center maintains a built-in regulatory apparatus for maintenance of "normal" temperature, and it is around this setpoint that mechanisms for heat production and heat conservation operate. The hypothalamus responds to the temperature of the blood which bathes the thermoreceptive areas of the brain, and also to signals arising from receptors in the periphery. This dual receptor system then regulates body heat gain or heat loss. The hypothalamus does not function until a threshold is reached, and then the response appears proportional to the input stimuli.[10] In some cases, the

[10]Hammel, H. T.: Regulation of internal body temperature. *Ann. Rev. Physiol.*, 30:641, 1968.

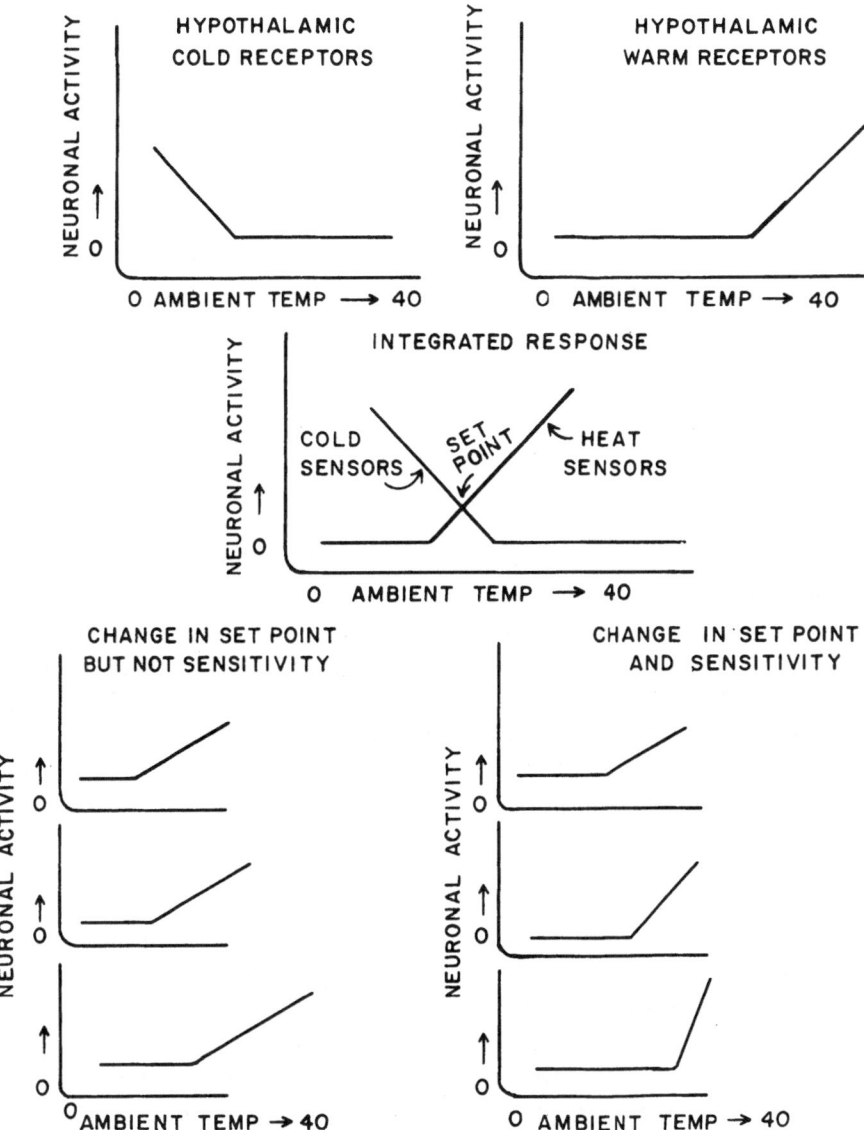

FIGURE 2.4: The neurophysiologic basis of temperature setpoint, represented by the sudden increase in neuronal activity (frequency of nerve firing) when setpoint is stimulated by alterations in ambient temperature. The slope of the response line determines sensitivity.

sensitivity of the response to the stimuli may be altered (change in sensitivity).

During cold exposure, sensory input from the peripheral cold receptors appears to alter setpoint or the threshold level for the effector response, but setpoint alterations do not significantly alter the proportional response which occurs once the setpoint temperature has been exceeded. Setpoint change does not necessarily alter sensitivity (the gain response), which is quite similar at all temperatures measured (Fig. 2.4). Besides the setpoint alterations with cold exposures, physiologic setpoint alterations occur with exercise, infection, drug administration, and electrolyte imbalance.

2.14   WHAT ARE THE MEDIATORS WHICH ALTER CENTRAL TEMPERATURE SETPOINT?

One hypothesis suggests that setpoint is regulated by a chemical thermostat, with setpoint determined by the relative levels of the neurohormones, norepinephrine, and 5-hydroxytryptamine. Stimuli which alter setpoint — blood temperature, pyrogens, drugs — do so by altering one of these two substances in relationship to the other.[11] The monoamine theory of temperature regulation has been tested in a variety of animals, and these studies demonstrate that neurohormones do alter body temperature and setpoint, but with great interspecies variation in the type of neurohormonal mediator that serves as the regulator, the dose response, and the effect produced (heat loss or heat gain). The chemical thermostat is thought to lie in the anterior hypothalamus, but the posterior thermoregulatory area is insensitive to application of monoamines and pyrogens. However, the posterior hypothalamus can alter setpoint when exposed to shifts in ionic balance. In the cat, elevations of extracellular sodium concentration above normal physiological concentrations within this region of the brain produced marked hyperthermia while an increase in calcium concentration caused hypothermia. Myers and Tytell have suggested that endotoxin-

---

[11] Feldberg, W., Hellon, R. F., and Myers, R. D.: Effect on temperature of monoamines injected into the cerebral ventricles of anesthetized dogs. *J. Physiol., 186*:416, 1966.

induced fever may arise from an endotoxin-induced alteration of ionic ratio within the hypothalamus.[12]

2.15   HOW DOES INFECTION STIMULATE INCREASED OXYGEN CONSUMPTION?

Infection causes a febrile response. This response results from blood-borne substances which cause a reset in the central temperature setpoint in the thermoregulatory center of the hypothalamus.

As previously noted, the thermoregulatory areas of the hypothalamus are concerned with heat dissipation and heat conservation. The biochemical messenger which arises during infection in the body is thought to reset the reference temperature in the hypothalamus upward. A normal temperature is interpreted by the temperature centers as cold, and the patient chills, even in a warm environment. Thus, the nervous system responds to increase body heat so the brain will be warmed to a new elevated setpoint temperature.

Two mechanisms are utilized to achieve an increased core temperature. *Vasoconstriction* limits heat loss from the body and increases body temperature; this is usually the first mechanism utilized by individuals who are in a warm or thermal neutral environment and develop a febrile response. *Increased heat production*, manifested by shivering and associated with increased oxygen consumption, may also occur, especially if the individual is exposed to a cool ambient temperature. Frequently, both of these mechanisms operate together to increase body heat and achieve a new setpoint temperature required by the brain.[13] Once this new reference temperature is achieved, temperature regulation will function to maintain this new level. The metabolic rate during this equilibration time (not during the phase of active shivering) should be accounted for by the Q_{10} effect.

When the infection clears, the setpoint returns to normal, and

[12]Myers, R. D., and Tyrell, M.: Fever: Reciprocal shift in brain sodium to calcium ratio as the set-point temperature rises. *Science, 178*:765, 1972.

[13]Buskirk, E. R., Thompson, R. H., Rubenstein, M., and Wolf, S. M.: Heat exchange in men and women following intravenous injection of endotoxin. *J. Appl. Physiol, 19*:907, 1964.

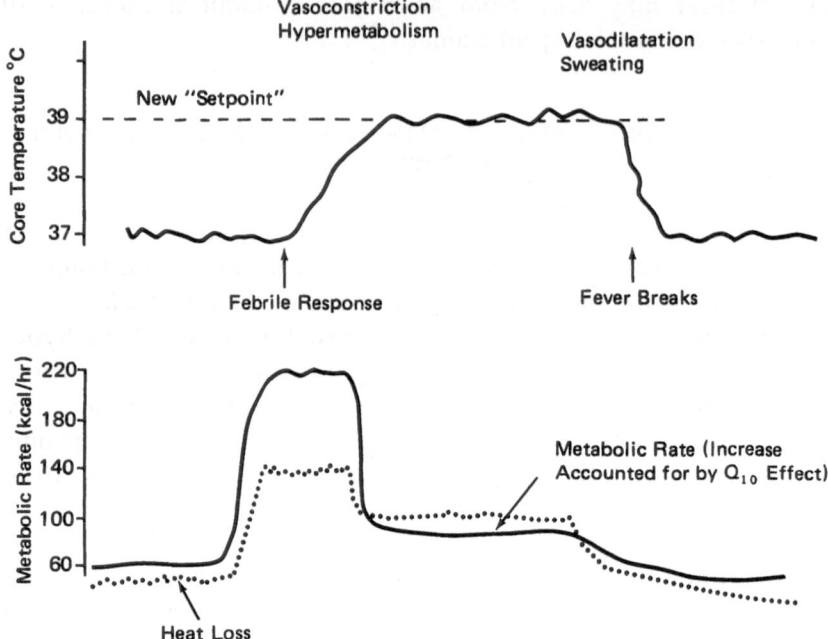

FIGURE 2.5: The response of body temperature, metabolic rate, and cutaneous heat loss
to a pyrogenic fever.

central nervous system mechanisms are activated to aid heat loss. Vasodilatation and sweating occur as body temperature falls and metabolic activity returns to a normal level. Thus, a new steady state is achieved, and skin and core temperatures are maintained around the new or "normal" setpoint.

2.16   WHAT ARE THE MEDIATORS OF THE FEBRILE RESPONSE TO INFECTION? WHAT IS ENDOGENOUS PYROGEN? HOW DOES IT DIFFER FROM EXOGENOUS OR BACTERIAL PYROGEN?

Filtrates of pus injected into animals cause elevation of body temperature. The substances which cause the pyrogenic reaction are lipopolysaccharides ("endotoxins") obtained from the cell wall of gram negative bacteria. These circulating factors act to alter host metabolic and physiologic responses following infection. However, products of the host's cells may serve as the afferent limb to the brain to stimulate fever. This concept gained support when Bennett and Beeson reported that a fever-inducing substance could be extracted from rabbit granulocytes.[14] Further studies revealed that the substance from granulocytes was regularly pyrogenic, while similar extracts from a wide variety of tissues carried no fever-inducing effect, and that the host pyrogen ("endogenous pyrogen") differed in many respects from the pyrogen of microbial origin.

A number of investigators have contributed to our knowledge of endogenous pyrogen, although the majority of the experimental work has been in animals. Tissue pyrogen may be activated by a variety of stimuli including exogenous pyrogen ("endotoxin"), viruses, bacteria, antigen–antibody complexes, and specific steroids. These stimulators cause a variety of cells to liberate endogenous pyrogen. Granulocytes were once thought to be the only cell type containing endogenous pyrogen, but later it was established that monocytes and macrophages – all cells capable of phagocytosis – also served as a pyrogen source. When stimulated, these cells produce and release a protein of 10,000–20,000 molecular weight which produces a prompt monophasic fever spike.[15] Partial species cross-reactivity to this substance has been observed but tolerance in the animal does not develop after repeated injections. In contrast, an animal becomes unresponsive or tolerant after repeated injections of "endotoxin" (exogenous pyrogen). The fever response to injection of endogenous pyrogen into the central nervous system is much greater than the response to a comparable intravenous dose. Although the presence and activity of tissue pyrogen have been demonstrated in man, repeated attempts to assay circulating pyrogen during high fevers have been unsuccessful, hampering definition of the specific role of tissue pyrogen in human infection and injury.

2.17   WHAT IS POSTTRAUMATIC FEVER? HOW SHOULD IT BE CONTROLLED?

When Cuthbertson first described the disturbance in nitrogen metabolism following long-bone fracture, he noted that all cases had an

---

[14]Bennett, I. L., and Beeson, P. B.: Studies on the pathogenesis of fever. I. The effect of injection of extracts and suspensions of uninfected rabbit tissue upon the body temperature of normal rabbits. *J. Exp. Med., 98:*477, 1953.

[15]Atkins, E., and Bodel, P.: Fever. *New Eng. J. Med., 286:*27, 1972.

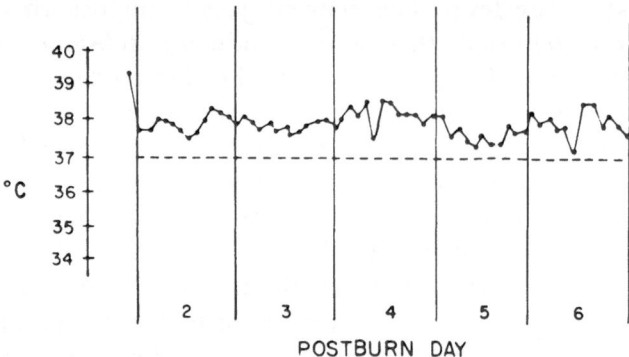

FIGURE 2.6: Rectal temperature in a 49-year-old male with a 68% total body surface burn demonstrates the persistent hyperpyrexia which occurs following injury.

associated fever but, with few exceptions, the temperature did not exceed 1–2°C above normal levels.[16] The increase in fever following injury was associated in the general time course with a rise in oxygen consumption and an increase in nitrogen excretion. This characteristic rise in core temperature which occurs following injury has been described as posttraumatic fever, and is an expected response to injury (Fig. 2.6).

Posttraumatic fever appears generally refractory to practical clinical methods of pharmacologic manipulation. In trauma patients, we accept a stable febrile course of up to 39°C and do not attempt to alter this fever. Constant surveillance for infection is required, and febrile spikes above 39°C or episodes of hypothermia with a sudden fall of core temperature below 37°C are often the first clinical indications of bacteremia. Treatment of traumatized or burn patients in a warm ambient environment will aid the maintenance of core temperature between 38 and 39°C and minimize the patients' energy expenditure and utilization of body stores for the generation of this additional heat. Supracaloric dietary support is required for maintenance of these febrile-injured patients in order to avoid disruption of lean body mass ("feed the fever").

[16]Cuthbertson, D. P.: The disturbance of metabolism produced by bony and non-bony injury, with notes of certain abnormal conditions of bone. *Biochem. J.*, *24*:1244, 1930.

2.18   WHAT OTHER DISEASE PROCESSES CAUSE FEVER?

In addition to a variety of infectious diseases, tissue damage and/or inflammation which cause fever, other disease processes have been associated with elevations in body temperature. Neoplastic disease can cause fever. Carcinoma of the stomach or pancreas with metastasis to the liver is usually associated with a temperature elevation and a febrile course may occur in patients with hypernephromas and the lymphoma group of neoplasms. Cancer patients should be carefully evaluated for the presence of infectious disease and multiple bacterial and fungal cultures obtained. Hematopoietic diseases (such as acute hemolytic episodes), vascular accidents, immune or allergic reactions (drug fevers), collagen diseases, and electrolyte imbalance (especially hypernatremia) are all associated with a febrile response.

2.19   SHOULD PATIENTS HAVE FEVER? WHEN SHOULD FEVER BE TREATED? HOW?

Fever is thought to be beneficial in a number of disease processes. The resistance to infection in experimental animals has been favorably influenced by raising the body temperature of the host animal.[17] In contrast, aged and debilitated people with infection, peritonitis, or injury frequently exhibit little or no pyrexia, and this is generally interpreted as a bad prognostic sign.

If the febrile response does not impose great discomfort on the patient, treatment is rarely necessary. In trauma patients, we support the hyperpyrexia by maintaining patients in a warm environment; a normal rectal temperature or hypothermia is usually an indication of gram-negative bacteremia. The febrile course during an infectious disease is a valuable indicator of the effect of treatment, and it is argued that antipyretics interfere with this clinical indicator and thus hamper use of core temperature as an accurate reflection of the course of the infection.

[17]Bernheim, H. A., and Kluger, M. J.: Fever: Effect of drug-induced antipyresis on survival. *Science, 193*:237, 1976.

There are situations when lowering of the body temperature is of vital importance, specifically during heat stroke, postoperative or interoperative hyperthermia, delirium or seizure activity associated with fever, and cardiocirculatory failure associated with hyperpyrexia. Use of antipyretics or other drugs which affect temperature setpoint, in addition to sponging the body surface with alcohol, increasing airflow over the surface, or utilizing cooling blankets to increase heat flow from the body are frequent techniques employed. Without pharmacologically altering setpoint, cooling the surface will stimulate additional vasoconstriction and heat production (through shivering). In cases of severe hyperthermia (>41°C) and vasoconstriction, rubbing the skin to promote vasodilatation or immersion of the patient into an ice bath should be considered life-saving.

2.20   WHAT IS THE RELATIONSHIP BETWEEN FEVER AND BODY CATABOLISM?

To distinguish the difference between the direct effects of infectious disease and the effect of increased tissue temperature on metabolism, Beisel and associates studied normal men placed in a hot chamber, adjusted to increase the subject's rectal temperature over 18 hr to 39.4°C, and maintained that temperature for 6 hr.[18] The adrenal responses and alterations in nitrogen metabolism during artificial hyperthermia resembled changes during infectious disease. Negative balance of nitrogen, potassium, and magnesium was produced by a combination of reduced dietary intake, increased urinary excretion, and increased sweat losses. With induced hyperthermia, there was greater electrolyte loss in sweat when compared to the hyperthermia of infectious disease, which does not cause these profound alterations in mineral metabolism.

2.21   WHAT IS THE RELATIONSHIP BETWEEN PULSE RATE AND FEVER?

With each 1°C rise in body temperature, there is an increase in pulse rate of approximately 10 beats/min (Fig. 2.7). Sturgis and

[18]Beisel, W. R., Goldman, R. F., and Joy, R. J. T.: Metabolic balance studies during induced hyperthermia in man. *J. Appl. Physiol.*, 24:1, 1968.

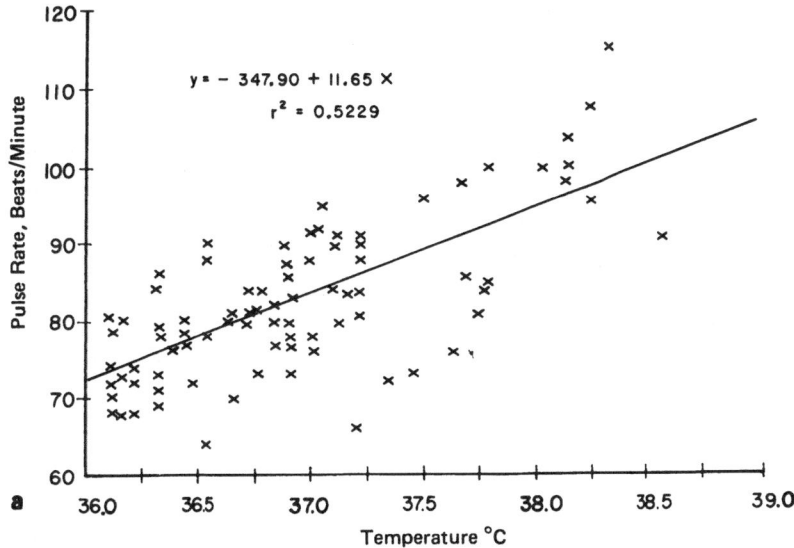

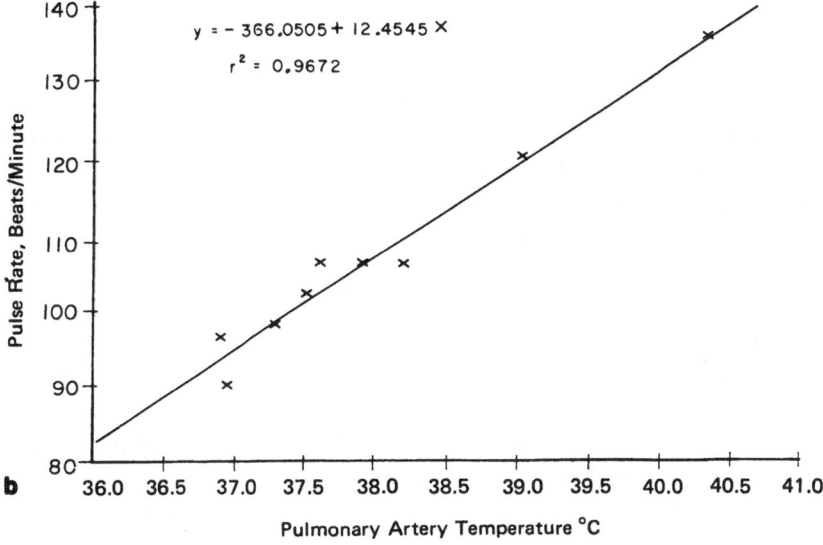

FIGURE 2.7: The relationship between body temperature (rectal or axillary) and pulse rate in patients with lower extremity injury (a), data from Cuthbertson. The response of heart rate and pulmonary artery temperature to rewarming a hypothermic injured patient (b). Data points observed at approximately 15-min intervals. Rectal temperatures slowly followed central vascular temperature.

Thomkins[19] related pulse rate to the extent of hyperthyroid hypermetabolism, and pointed out that the rapidity of the heart rate is perhaps the best guide for treating this condition. They found a close relationship between pulse rate and basal metabolism in the majority of the hyperthyroid patients and rarely found the pulse rate at complete rest to be below 90 beats/min in patients with basal metabolic rates greater than +15. Hypermetabolism was quite rare in patients with a pulse rate below 80. Whether this is due to concomitant effects of the thyroid gland on the cardiovascular system and on metabolism or a response of the cardiovascular system to the increased heat load has not been clearly demonstrated.

2.22   WHAT DRUGS AFFECT TEMPERATURE SETPOINT?

A wide variety of substances have been injected into the hypothalamus in the laboratory animal to demonstrate pharmacologic influences on temperature regulation. However, these experiments are of little value to the clinician unless systemic administration of the drug will affect temperature setpoint.

Although salicylates are the common antipyretic administered in febrile man, their method of action is still unknown. Salicylates are effective in attenuating or eliminating the fever resulting from a systemic injection of bacterial or leukocyte pyrogen. As previously mentioned, Myers has suggested that salicylate effect in the central nervous system may be due to alterations of the ionic balance across the cell membrane in the hypothalamic area. Other salicylate-like antipyretics are acetaminophen, phenacetin, antipyrine, and aminopyrine.

Some general anesthetics have a pronounced effect in diminishing sympathetic outflow from the central nervous system. This effect is usually ascribed to the nonspecific depression of the central nervous system by the agent rather than to selective action of thermal regulatory centers. However, the attendant hypothermia which frequently accompanies major operations is due in part to the decreased heat production that occurs secondary to general

---

[19]Sturgis, C. C., and Thompkins, E. H.: Study of the correlation of basal metabolism and pulse rate in patients with hypermetabolism. *Arch. Intern. Med.*, 26:467, 1920.

anesthesia. Increased heat loss also occurs in patients undergoing operations in the cool environment of the operating room.

Morphine has a pronounced effect on decreasing heat production, which may be associated with a fall in body temperature. Although small doses of morphine exert minimal effects on heat production and heat loss, morphine, given in an anesthetic dose in the operating room or in repeated dosages to patients on a ventilator, may have a pronounced effect on sympathetic outflow from the brain and greatly diminish heat production (Fig. 2.8). Similarly chlorpromazine and some other tranquilizers may cause a fall in heat production, while amphetamine may cause an increase in oxygen

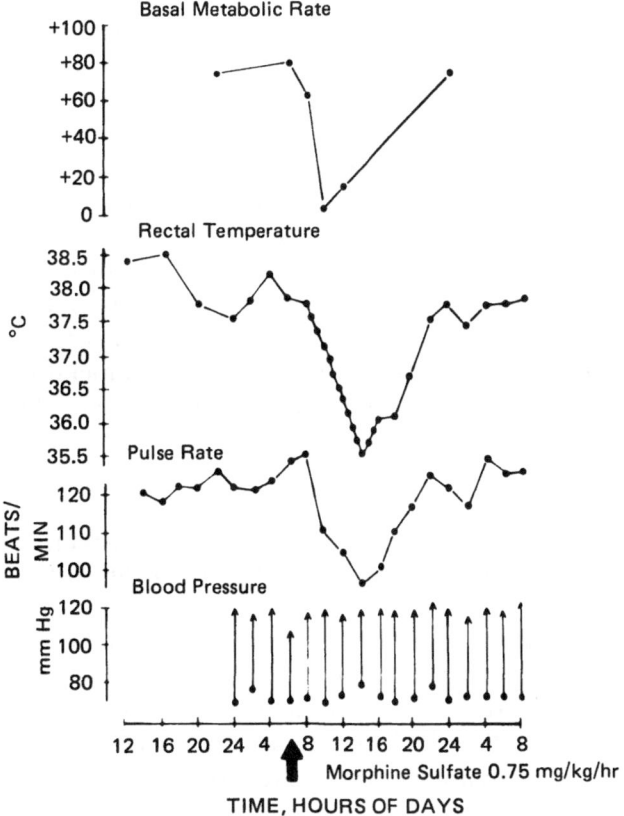

FIGURE 2.8: The effect of morphine anesthesia on metabolic rate, pulse, and rectal temperature; administered to a 21-year-old male with 83% total body surface burn. Blood pressure and arterial oxygen content were unchanged throughout the study.

consumption, resulting mainly from an increase in central nervous system activity rather than direct stimulation of the thermal regulatory areas. Other commonly used drugs are thought to affect central setpoint.[20] L-Dopa caused a slight reduction in core temperature in some normal men studied in a cool room. Atropine diminishes the rate of sweating and in large doses causes hyperthermia, yet atropine may affect central thermal regulatory areas, resulting in a decrease in heat production.

2.23 WHY DO PATIENTS BECOME HYPOTHERMIC IN THE OPERATING ROOM?

Man responds to cold exposure by peripheral vasoconstriction and hypermetabolism (primarily shivering). Both of these compensatory mechanisms are depressed or eliminated by most general anesthetics, which cause cutaneous vasodilatation and abolish muscle movement. Muscle relaxants also prevent shivering. Patients in the operating room are extremely vulnerable to increased heat loss and may become hypothermic in cold operating theaters if large volumes of cold iv fluids are administered or if wounds or body cavities are irrigated with cool solutions (Fig. 2.9). Lightly anesthetized, paralyzed, adult patients undergoing operation in rooms warmer than 21°C remained normothermic.[21] This ambient temperature should even be much warmer when operating on babies, thermally injured patients, or septic hypothermic individuals.

2.24 HOW DO ELECTROLYTES ALTER BODY TEMPERATURE? WHAT HORMONES AFFECT TEMPERATURE SETPOINT?

Dehydration in infants is usually associated with a febrile response, once referred to as "inanition fever." The febrile response is greater if the dehydrated patient is hypertonic (i.e., hypernatremic). Moyer reproduced this finding in rats and found a decrease in oxygen consumption with hypo-osmolar dehydration, a marked rise in

[20]Lomax, P.: Drugs and body temperature. *Int. Rev. Neurobiol.*, *12*:1, 1970.
[21]Morris, R. H.: Influence of ambient temperature on patient temperature during intraabdominal surgery. *Ann. Surg.*, *173*:230, 1971.

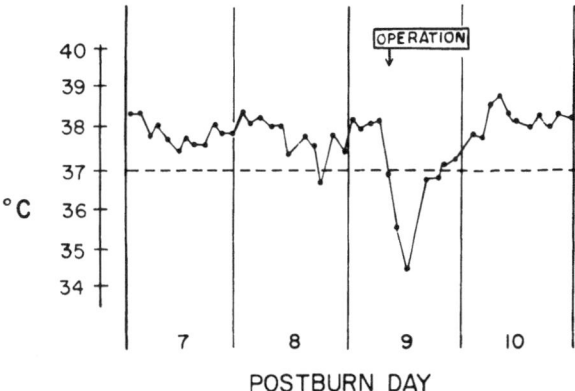

POSTBURN DAY

FIGURE 2.9: Hypothermia accompanying general anesthesia. Rectal temperature was monitored in this 49-year-old male with a 68% total body surface burn undergoing debridement of his burn wound.

oxygen consumption during hyperosmolar dehydration, and no change in metabolic rate during isotonic dehydration.[22] This effect may be mediated by the central nervous system, for injection of sodium into the thermoregulatory center causes a prompt rise in body temperature. A similar association between oxygen consumption and extracellular sodium concentration has been observed *in vitro*, presumably through the stimulation of the Na–K cell pump that is augmented by the increased sodium concentration in the medium.[23]

A number of hormones stimulate calorigenesis, and their feedback signal to the hypothalamus is thought to be indirect: these substances apparently do not cross the blood–brain barrier to affect the hypothalamus directly. Prostaglandins are substances which cause fever, but this characteristic response is observed only with the hypothalamic injection of PGE_1, and not the other prostaglandin compounds. The effect of PGE_1 on thermal regulation is thought to alter temperature setpoint and not thermal sensitivity.[24] Aspirin

[22]Moyer, C. A., and Nissan, S.: Alterations in the basal oxygen consumption of rats attendant upon three types of dehydration. *Ann. Surg., 154*:51, 1961.

[23]Nissan, S., Aviram, A., Czaczkes, J. W., Ullmann, L., and Ullmann, T. D.: Increased O_2 consumption of the rat diaphragm by elevated NaCl concentrations. *Amer. J. Physiol., 210*:1222, 1966.

[24]Stitt, J. T., Hardy, J. D., and Stolwijk, J. A. J.: PGE_1 fever: Its effect on thermal regulation at different low ambient temperatures. *Amer. J. Physiol, 227*:622, 1974.

blocks prostaglandin synthesis and this is one mechanism postulated for the antipyretic effect of salicylates. The role of prostaglandins in clinical fever is not known.

2.25 HOW IS TEMPERATURE CONTROL RELATED TO METABOLIC CONTROL?

Intimately involved with the hypothalamic centers controlling body temperature are areas that regulate food intake and substrate flow. The role of the central nervous system in metabolic control was first demonstrated by Claude Bernard in 1849, when he reported the appearance of glucosuria following puncture of the fourth ventricle in dogs. The studies of Cannon emphasized the role of the sympathetic nervous system and adrenal medulla in the defense reaction of the body.

Central to hypothalamic control of metabolism and temperature is the function of the ventral medial and ventral lateral nuclei of the hypothalamus, which are important for regulation of food intake, substrate flow, and heat production.[25] The first experimental evidence for this association was presented by Hetherington and Ransom,[26] who reported that bilateral destruction of the ventromedial hypothalamus of the rat resulted in hyperphagia and massive obesity. Later, it was found that destructive lesions of the ventrolateral nucleus of the hypothalamus resulted in reduction or a cessation of food intake. The ventromedial nucleus was labeled the "satiety center" and the ventrolateral area the "feeding center," and the presence of nerve fibers between these two regulatory areas, presumably for transmission of inhibitory signals from the satiety or feeding centers, was demonstrated. Therefore, destruction of the ventromedial nucleus (satiety center) removes inhibition on the feeding center (ventrolateral nucleus), resulting in hyperphagia. Stimulation of the ventromedial nucleus produces the opposite effect.

The first control mechanism of blood glucose, substrate flow,

[25]Frohman, L. A.: The hypothalamus and metabolic control. *In* H. L. Ioachim (Ed.): *Pathobiology Annual.* New York, 1971, p. 353.
[26]Hetherington, A. W., and Ransom, S. W.: Hypothalamic lesions and adiposity in the rat. *Anat. Rec.*, 78:149, 1940.

and heat production is thought to reside in the hypothalamus and involves both sympathetic and parasympathetic stimulation. The sympathetic pathways travel from the ventromedial nucleus of the hypothalamus (from the sympathetic center of the brain) by way of the floor of the fourth ventricle to sympathetic fibers in the spinal cord, then to splanchnic nerves of the liver, pancreas, and adrenal gland. Activation of this system results in glycogenolysis and increased glucose entry into the circulation. The parasympathetic component originates from the ventrolateral nucleus and, when stimulated, increases glycogen synthetase activity of the liver and provides a hormonal environment favoring glucose storage.

2.26   IS THERE EVIDENCE FOR ALTERED HYPOTHALAMIC FUNCTION FOLLOWING STRESS?

Alterations in hypothalamic function have been demonstrated in both animals and man during stress, infection, and following injury. Animals subjected to high environmental temperature, muscle exercise, or mild electric shock increase their turnover of brain norepinephrine and increase body temperature. In the rat, norepinephrine turnover in the hypothalamus is increased for prolonged periods after extreme muscular exertion. Injury alters monoamine concentrations in the rat hypothalamus and hind limb ischemia lowers the threshold for the onset of shivering induced by preoptic cooling.[27]

In man, increased evidence is accumulating that the metabolic alterations after injury result from homeostatic readjustment within the hypothalamus. ACTH and HGH elaboration occurs in response to a wide variety of stresses, including injury, infection, hemorrhage, and operation. The same hormonal response occurs during defense reactions initiated by electrical stimulation of the hypothalamus in rhesus monkeys. The ACTH and HGH response can be blocked in man at the hypothalamic level by morphine anesthesia. HGH levels are elevated following thermal injury in spite of associated hyperglycemia.[28] However, a diminished HGH response occurs to pro-

[27]Stoner, H. B.: Effects of injury on the responses to thermal stimulation of the hypothalamus. *J. Appl. Physiol., 33*:665, 1972.

[28]Wilmore, D. W., Orcutt, T. W., Mason, A. D., Jr., and Pruitt, B. A., Jr.: Alterations in hypothalamic function following thermal injury. *J. Trauma, 15*:697, 1975.

vocative stimuli of insulin hypoglycemia and arginine hydrochloride infusion during the acute phase of injury when compared with the response observed in convalescent patients or normal man.

2.27   DOES THE ALTERED HYPOTHALAMIC FUNCTION IN STRESSED MAN AFFECT THERMOREGULATION?

Altered thermal regulation occurs in injured man. Average core temperature of burn patients is elevated above normal and mean skin temperature is also increased in all ambient temperatures studied when compared to normal man, demonstrating that burn patients are internally warm, not externally cold.[29] Burn patients studied in a warm environment remained hypermetabolic, and demonstrated elevated core and skin temperatures. Heat production did not return to normal levels in the warm environment, and increased oxygen consumption observed in such patients could not be accounted for by increased tissue temperature (Q_{10} effect).

The reset in metabolic activity appeared to be related to adjustments of central temperature setpoint. Burn patients placed in an environmental control chamber were allowed to regulate their own ambient temperature to achieve comfort, using a bedside remote control unit. The mean ambient temperature selected for comfort was significantly increased compared to normal man and was generally related to the size of the injury. When comfortable, the burn patients had a significantly higher core and mean skin temperature than the normals. Reset or readjustment in hypothalamic temperature setpoint following injury is suggested by the fact that burn patients felt comfortable at elevated ambient temperatures which were uncomfortable for normal man (Table 2.5). Moreover, the patients maintained elevated core and skin temperatures while subjectively comfortable, similar to the central temperature readjustment that occurs during the febrile response to infection.

[29]Wilmore, D. W., Long, J. M., Mason, A. D., Jr., Skreen, R. W., and Pruitt, B. A., Jr.: Catecholamines: Mediator of the hypermetabolic response to thermal injury. *Ann. Surg.*, *180*:653, 1974.

Table 2.5   Ambient Temperatures of Comfort (Mean ± SE)

	N	Room comfort temperature (°C)	T_{skin} (°C)	T_{core} (°C)
Control	5	27.8 ± 0.6	33.4 ± 0.6	36.9 ± 0.1
Burn patients[a]	9	30.4 ± 0.7 $p < 0.05$	35.2 ± 0.4 $p < 0.05$	38.4 ± 0.3 $p < 0.01$

[a]Mean burn size 39% total body surface.

2.28   WHAT STIMULATES THE HYPOTHALAMUS TO PRODUCE "POSTTRAUMATIC FEVER"?

The quickest route for signaling the brain that tissue injury has occurred is by sensory nerves, and the importance of the afferent nervous signals to the hypothalamus has been well described following pain, hypoxia, hypotension and hypovolemia. Afferent nervous signals are essential for the immediate release of ACTH and ADH following stress. During the flow phase of injury, an intact brain stem is necessary for a posttraumatic response, but denervation of the wound or interruption of the sensory input to the brain does not appear to diminish the hypermetabolic response to thermal injury (Table 2.7). Alterations in albumin turnover have been observed in paraplegic patients following operations on the denervated lower extremity, supporting the thesis that circulating factors provide the afferent limb signals to the brain, resulting in a reset in metabolic activity.[30]

2.29   HOW IS BLOOD GLUCOSE RELATED TO BODY TEMPERATURE AND HEAT PRODUCTION?

Insulin-induced hypoglycemia causes a fall in body temperature.[31] This response appears to be the direct result of glucose deprivation of

[30]Davies, J. W. L., Liljedahl, S.-O., and Reizenstein, R. R.: Metabolic studies with labelled albumin in patients with paraplegia and other injuries. *Injury, 1*:271, 1970.
[31]Molnar, G. W., and Read, R. C.: Hypoglycemia and body temperature. *J. Am. Med. Assoc., 227*:916, 1974.

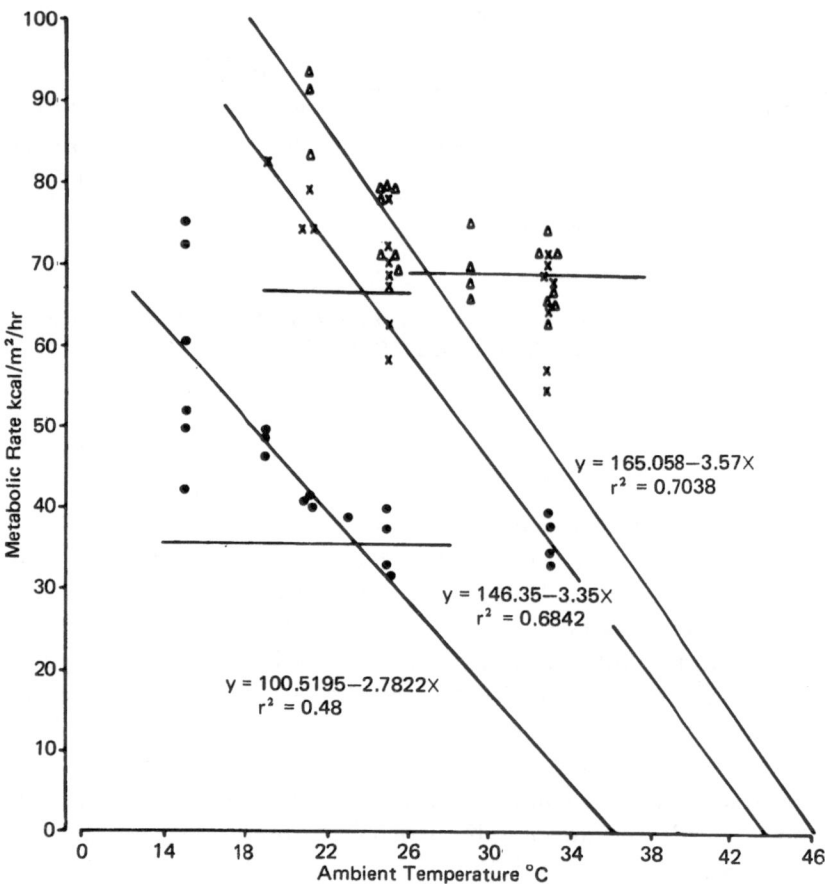

FIGURE 2.10: Heat production in response to alterations in ambient temperature was assessed in normals and in thermally injured patients. The horizontal lines represent the mean of the lowest level of heat production that could be obtained for each group of individuals during the study. As ambient temperature is lowered, metabolic rate increases and these measurements above basal have been fitted to a regression line. The slope of the line reflects body insulation and the point where it crosses the horizontal bar determines the "critical temperature." The intercept of these lines with the X-axis is thought to reflect central temperature setpoints or thermal drives of these individuals. Note the apparent increase in temperature setpoint in the burn patients when compared to the normals (Table 2.6). • Controls, x Burns 35–50%, △ Burns >60%.

Table 2.6   Analysis of Critical Temperature Curves

	Controls	Burns 35–50% TBS	Burns > 60% TBS
Basal metabolic rate			
($kcal/m^2/hr$)	36.0	66.9	69.3
$T_{Critical}$ (°C)	23.2	23.7	26.8
Slope	2.78	3.33	3.57
$T_{Intercept}$ (°C)	36.1	43.7	46.2

Table 2.7   The Effect of CNS Injury and Afferent Nervous Blockade on
Posttraumatic Hypermetabolism (Mean, Range, or ± SE)

CNS injury	N	Burn size (% BSA^a)	Age (years)	Postburn day studied	Metabolic rate ($kcal/m^2/hr$) Measured	Metabolic rate ($kcal/m^2/hr$) Predicted from burn size
Cerebral contusion	1	26	15	15	65.6	53.0
Cerebral contusion	1	48	23	8	88.2	68.0
Cerebral contusion (T-11 spinal cord transection)	1	60^b	27	3	92.0	74.4
Cerebral edema (flat EEG)	1	23	19	3	30.8	56.1
Afferent nervous blockade					Before	After
Topical anesthesia to burn wound	3	66 (53–78.5)	28 (25–30)	13 (10–17)	77.8 ± 4.2	77.5 ± 2.5
Spinal anesthesia	1	33^c	39	33	57.3	63.8

^{a}BSA = body surface area.
^{b}Burn over lower trunk and lower extremities.
^{c}Multiple fractures and burns of lower extremities.

the thermoregulating neurons of the hypothalamus rather than the
lack of available body fuel for generating heat.[32] Hypothermia can
be induced by hypothalamic injection of 2-deoxy-D-glucose, a
glucose analogue which blocks intracellular glucose utilization
causing intracellular hypoglycemia. The febrile response in animals

[32]Freinkel, N., Metzger, B. E., Harris, E., Robinson, S., and Mager, M.: The hypothermia of
hypoglycemia. New Eng. J. Med., 287:841, 1972.

following PGE_1 administration and yeast fever is blocked or attenuated following hypothalamic glucose blockade, demonstrating the dependency of the thermoregulatory centers on glucose.[33]

Hyperglycemia may occur during episodes of hyperthermia. Increased mass flow of glucose from the liver to peripheral tissue results from the sympathoadrenal response stimulated by the alteration in temperature setpoint. The interrelationship between increased mass flow of substrate and increased heat production is discussed in a later section (see p. 165).

2.30   WHAT IS HEAT EXHAUSTION? ... HEAT STROKE? HOW ARE THE HEAT OVERLOAD SYNDROMES TREATED?

Acute hyperpyrexia is associated with hard physical work in a hot, moist ambient environment[34] or occurs in elderly individuals with preexisting diseases such as alcoholism, heart disease, or obesity who are exposed to hot temperatures. The physiological disturbances may be classified as:

1. *Heat cramps*: acute salt depletion
2. *Heat exhaustion*: water depletion and hypovolemia manifesting symptoms of headache, vomiting, tachycardia, and hypotension
3. *Heat stroke*: severe CNS disturbance, hyperpyrexia ($>41°C$ rectal), and hot, dry skin.

Sweating usually stops before the onset of heat stroke, demonstrating profound homeostatic dysfunction in these hyperpyrexic individuals. Heat-unloading and support of vital organ systems are the priorities of treatment. The patient should be cooled by any means, preferably in an ice bath. Phenothiazine may be administered to reduce shivering if it occurs. Cautious administration of a balanced salt solution (rarely more than 1400 ml in the first 4 hr) replenishes fluid and electrolyte deficits, providing circulatory support. Digitalis should be administered in the presence of heart failure and isoproterenol infused for treatment of hypotension to restore a high

[33]Robinson, S., and Mager, M.: 2-Deoxy-D-glucose inhibition of prostaglandin E_1 hyperthermia and yeast fever in mice. *J. Appl. Physiol.*, *38*:1092, 1975.

[34]Clowes, G. H. A., Jr., and O'Donnell, T. F.: Heat stroke. *New Eng. J. Med.*, 291:564, 1974.

cardiac output. Adequate circulatory function is essential in these patients in order to transport heat loads from the core to the surface for heat exchange. Mannitol is administered to promote urinary output and ventilatory support utilized as indicated. Disseminated intravascular coagulation has been observed in heat stroke patients and is effectively treated by systemic heparinization.

2.31 WHAT IS THE ROLE OF PHYSICAL ACTIVITY AND DEHYDRATION IN OVERHEATING?

Heavy work in a warm environment places extreme demands on circulation for (1) nutrient supply to the muscle mass, and (2) simultaneous maintenance of heat flow to the surface to facilitate heat transfer. Blood flow to muscle to satisfy local nutrient requirements has priority over circulation to the skin to facilitate heat transfer. Progressive dehydration in the face of increasing work loads and rising body temperature further compromises sweating. Blood flow to the skin is reduced while muscle nutrient flow is favored, placing no immediate limitation on work capacity; thus, the individual frequently continues to work until heat exhaustion or heat stroke occurs.

2.32 WHAT ARE THE SYMPTOMS AND TREATMENT OF MALIGNANT HYPERTHERMIA WHICH OCCURS DURING ANESTHESIA?

Unexplained tachycardia and tachypnea during anesthesia associated with a $0.5°C$ temperature rise may be the first signs of malignant hyperthermia which occurs under anesthesia. The apparent uncontrolled rise in body temperature (often above $41°C$) is associated with metabolic acidosis, hyperkalemia, altered coagulation, and frequently with muscle rigidity.

The treatment of the patient with a rising body temperature of this magnitude must be rapid and heroic. The patient should be placed on an ice blanket and packed in ice. Refrigerated intravenous solutions are administered and body cavities (pleural and peritoneal, if open), stomach, and bladder are lavaged with cold solutions. Cardiopulmonary bypass as a method for rapid heat exchange has been utilized in patients refractory to usual therapy. Other supportive techniques include administration of sodium bicarbonate, insulin and glucose, chlorpromazine, and mannitol.

The etiology of malignant hyperpyrexia is not completely known, but this response to general anesthesia is observed in families and thought to be related to an inherited error in calcium metabolism that resides in the muscle cell.[35]

The muscle rigor may be triggered by specific anesthetic agents, particularly succinylcholine and/or halothane. Dramatic reduction in heat production has been observed following administration of procainamide or procaine, which is thought to reverse the elevated calcium level in the cytoplasm by calcium uptake by the sacroplasmic reticulum of the muscle cell.

2.33   WHAT CAUSES ACCIDENTAL HYPOTHERMIA? HOW IS IT TREATED?

Accidental hypothermia is occasionally observed in individuals exposed to cold ambient air or submerged in cold water. It most commonly occurs in the very young or elderly patient. The thermoregulatory mechanisms in thermally neutral and cold environments are significantly affected by age. Young men rapidly react to cold stress by increasing their metabolic rates and minimizing peripheral heat loss by rapid cutaneous vasoconstriction. Older men do not increase heat production to the same extent and are less able to maintain body heat stores by vasoconstriction.[36] Infants are compromised by the increased ratio of surface area to body mass which potentiates heat loss. Undernutrition and associated infection are frequently related factors which occur in hypothermic patients.[37] Severe myxedema has also been associated with a pronounced fall in body temperature.

Treatment is initiated by gradual rewarming, maintenance of adequate cardiocirculatory function, respiratory support, infusion of

[35]Gordon, R. A., Britt, B. A., and Kalow, W.: *International Symposium on Malignant Hyperthermia.* Springfield, Ill., Charles C Thomas, 1973.

[36]Wagner, J. A., Robinson, S., and Marino, R. P.: Age and temperature regulation of humans in neutral and cold environments. *J. Appl. Physiol., 37:*562, 1974.

[37]Arneil, G. C., and Kerr, M. M.: Severe hypothermia in Glasgow infants in winter. *Lancet,* 2:756, 1963.

glucose, and correction of acid—base and electrolyte disturbances. Death results from ventricular fibrillation which usually occurs at core temperatures below 28°C and is associated with heart disease, hypoxia, or acidosis. Shivering should be permitted in patients whose thermoregulatory mechanisms are perfectly normal. However, temperature control is markedly reduced at 25°C, and some external heating is necessary to bring the core temperature to 30—32°C; then spontaneous rewarming is allowed.[38] Rapid rewarming is advocated by some but may be associated with severe shock and circulatory failure. Constant temperature monitoring is essential, using indwelling thermal probes. (Note that most commonly used clinical thermometers do not measure temperatures below 94° F or 35°C.)

2.34   HOW DOES ALCOHOL CAUSE HYPOTHERMIA?

Alcohol is frequently a causal agent in the elderly patient who sustains accidental hypothermia. Alcohol causes vasodilatation and suppresses shivering, thereby increasing heat loss and decreasing heat production during cold exposure.

Alcohol blocks hepatic gluconeogenesis, resulting in diminished glucose flow from the liver to peripheral tissue and hypoglycemia.[39] The hypoglycemia is potentiated if the subject has been exercising or is partially or totally fasted. Thus, an unconscious hypothermic patient may be somnolent not because of excess alcohol ingestion but because of hypoglycemia.

2.35   WHY DO PATIENTS WITH GRAM-NEGATIVE INFECTION BECOME HYPOTHERMIC?

Hypothermia is frequently associated with gram-negative bacteremia. Peripheral vasodilatation promotes increased heat loss from infected patients and alters heat balance. However, gram-negative infection blunts hepatic gluconeogenesis that may be a primary mechanism for

[38]Blair, E.: *Clinical Hypothermia.* New York, McGraw-Hill, 1964, p. 183.
[39]Frenkel, N., Arky, R. A., Singer, D. L., Cohen, A. K., Bleicher, S. J., Anderson, J. B., Silbert, C. K., and Foster, A. E.: Alcohol hypoglycemia. IV. Current concepts of its pathogenesis. *Diabetes, 14*:350, 1965.

heat production in traumatized patients. Diminished hepatic gluconeogenesis and hypoglycemia have been associated with overwhelming infection and have been observed in septic injured patients.[40] The fall in glucose mass flow from liver to the peripheral tissues is related to the decrease in oxygen consumption and a fall in core temperature.

Thus, patients with gram-negative sepsis may have increased heat loss and an associated decrease in heat production, both of which contribute to the progressive fall in body temperature.

[40]Wilmore, D. W., Mason, A. D., Jr., and Pruitt, B. A., Jr.: Impaired glucose flow in burned patients with gram-negative sepsis. *Surg. Gynecol. Obstet., 143*:720, 1976.

CHAPTER 3

Hormonal Control of Body Fuels

3.1 WHAT ARE HORMONES?

The name "hormone," derived from the Greek root meaning to excite, arouse, or set in motion, was proposed by Starling to describe chemical agents which are released from one group of cells, travel by the blood stream, and affect other cell populations. Huxley placed less emphasis on the mode of travel of these substances and suggested that the prime role of hormones is to *transfer information* from one set of cells to another, to evoke a response beneficial for the cell population as a whole.

Recent advances in hormonal assay, particularly with the development of immunoassay techniques for quantification of small peptide molecules, allow changes in the level of specific "information transfer units" — hormones — to be related to specific stimuli evoked by alterations in the external environment or the internal milieu. Additional studies designed to evaluate the effect of hormonal administration or hormone blockade have further characterized the biochemical and biophysical alterations which are set in motion by hormonal mediators.

3.2   WHAT ARE THE STORAGE HORMONES? WHAT ARE THEIR EFFECTS? WHAT ARE THE MOBILIZING HORMONES?

Insulin is the principal storage hormone and promotes the movement and storage of metabolic fuels within cells. This effect is augmented by several other hormones (Fig. 3.1) and the parasympathetic nervous system, but insulin plays the dominant role in converting body substrate to storage fuels. In the nonstress state, insulin responds to blood glucose concentrations to facilitate glucose entry into many tissues. Insulin also facilitates lipogenesis and membrane transport of amino acids. Insulin deficiency or insulin lack results in mobilization of storage fuels and body wasting.

Mobilization of peripheral fuels is greatly enhanced by sympathetic nervous system discharge and catecholamine elaboration. Insulin deficiency and catecholamine elaboration appear to exert a complementary or additive effect in body fuel mobilization. Other hormones exert effects on key metabolic pathways and their participation in substrate mobilization or storage is summarized in Fig. 3.1.

3.3   HOW IS INSULIN STORED?...RELEASED? WHAT IS THE HALF-LIFE OF INSULIN?

The protein molecule insulin is synthesized in the beta pancreatic cell as a single chain precursor, proinsulin. This molecule is then broken

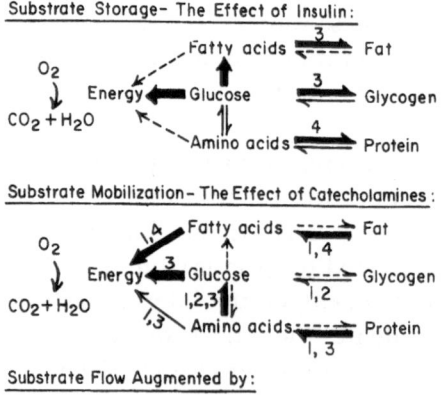

FIGURE 3.1: The effect of hormones on substrate storage and mobilization. Adapted from Bondy, P. K.: Disorders of carbohydrate metabolism. *In: Diseases of Metabolism.* Philadelphia, W. B. Saunders, 1969, p. 220.

and forms the active protein hormone which contains two peptide chains joined by two disulfide bridges of cystine. About 200 units of insulin are stored in the granules of the beta cell of the pancreas; only 40–60 units are required daily. The insulin stores in the pancreas decrease with age and vary with the quantity of carbohydrate in the diet. Pancreatic insulin content markedly decreases with starvation. Dietary factors are standardized before a glucose tolerance test by ensuring adequate carbohydrate intake for several days before the test.

Insulin is released from the beta cells into the portal venous blood which exposes the liver to high insulin concentrations. Normal metabolism and replication of the hepatocyte may be dependent on the high portal concentrations of insulin.[1] Studies of endogenously secreted and exogenously administered labeled insulin indicate that approximately 50% of the insulin in the portal system is degraded by the liver during a single passage through the portal system.[2] The remaining insulin that passes through the liver exerts its effect on peripheral tissue; the concentration of insulin measured in peripheral blood is a reflection of the quantity of insulin that is not degraded in the liver. In some patients with liver disease, hepatic extraction of insulin may be diminished and an increased quantity of insulin may reach the periphery when compared to normals.

Studies of labeled insulin demonstrate that the hormone molecule is removed from the blood stream quite rapidly and the half-life appears to be less than 10 min.[3] Thus, insulin is most effective if administered either subcutaneously or intramuscularly, or if given in a constant intravenous infusion, utilizing a syringe pump, rather than by periodic intravenous injections of regular insulin.

3.4   HOW IS INSULIN MEASURED? HOW IS THE INSULIN RESPONSE TO GLUCOSE ASSESSED?

Insulin assay, which was once dependent on biological responses for quantification, has been revolutionized by the development of

[1] Starzl, T. E., Porter, K. A., and Putnam, C. W.: Intraportal insulin protects from the liver injury of portacaval shunt in dogs. *Lancet,* 2:1241, 1975.

[2] Samols, E., and Ryder, J. A.: Studies on tissue uptake of insulin in man using a differential immunoassay for endogenous and exogenous insulin. *J. Clin. Invest.,* 40:2092, 1961.

[3] Tomasi, T., Sledz, D., Wales, J. K., and Recant, L.: Insulin half-life in normal and diabetic subjects. *Proc. Soc. Exp. Biol., 126*:315, 1967.

radioimmunoassay techniques. Yalow and Berson utilized the antigenic properties of insulin to develop specific antibodies.[4] Utilizing the technique of competitive binding of labeled and unlabeled insulin by the specific antibodies, multiple samples for insulin can now be rapidly and economically analyzed.

Insulin can be related to blood glucose in the basal state or its time course and response determined following a provocative challenge, usually utilizing glucose for stimulation. Basal insulin may be ratioed to the glucose level (expressed as units of insulin/blood glucose, mg/100 ml) to determine if the basal or unstimulated insulin level is appropriate for the measured blood glucose concentration (Table 3.1). The insulin response to a glucose load is classically

Table 3.1   Basal and Stimulated Insulin Concentrations Following Glucose Administration in Normals and Acutely Injured Patients (Mean ± SE)

	Normals	Burn shock
Number of studies	12	4
Fasting insulin (μU/ml)	22 ± 3	20 ± 6
Fasting glucose (mg/100 ml)	85 ± 3	149 ± 17
$\dfrac{\text{Fasting insulin } (\mu U/ml)}{\text{Fasting glucose } (mg/100 \text{ ml})} \times 100$	24 ± 2	13 ± 4
0–10′ Δ insulin	58 ± 13	10 ± 6
$\dfrac{\text{0–10′ insulin area}}{\text{0–10′ glucose area}}$	0.36 ± 0.07	0.15 ± 0.07
$\dfrac{\text{Total insulin area}}{\text{Total glucose area}}$	0.48 ± 0.10	0.21 ± 0.15

assessed by determining the insulinogenic index described by Seltzer.[5] This index is the ratio of the area under the insulin curve above basal, divided by the area under the glucose curve above basal: or the insulin response divided by the physiologic stimulus (Fig. 3.2). Lerner has emphasized that the major quantity of insulin release occurs immediately following the provocative stimulus and suggests

[4]Yalow, R. S., and Berson, S. A.: Immunoassay of endogenous plasma insulin in man. *J. Clin. Invest., 39:*1157, 1960.

[5]Seltzer, H. S., Allen, E. W., Herron, A. L., and Brennan, M. T.: Insulin secretion in response to glycemic stimulus: relation of delayed initial release to carbohydrate intolerance in mild diabetes mellitus. *J. Clin. Invest., 46:*323, 1967.

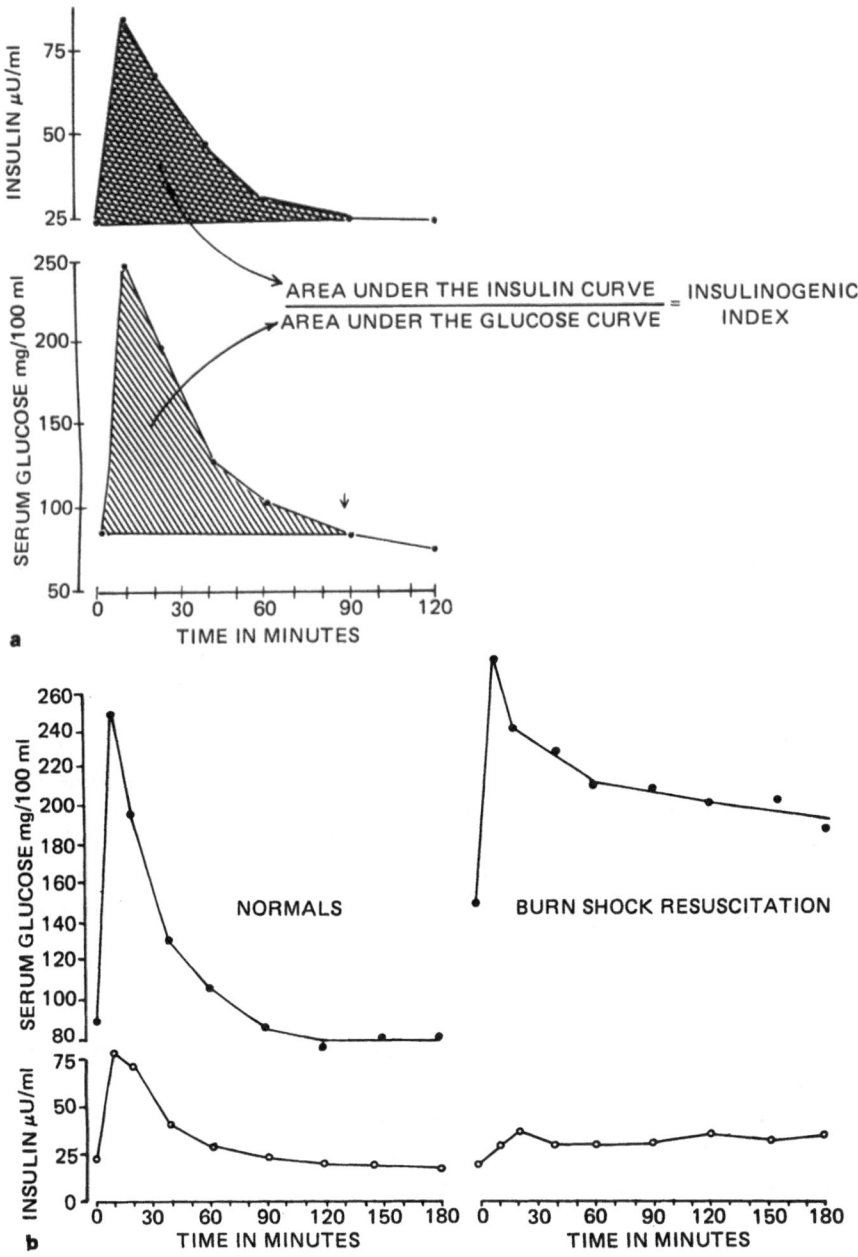

FIGURE 3.2: (a) The shaded areas represent the cumulative enhancement of serum glucose concentration above the fasting value (bottom curve) and the corresponding increases of insulin above basal. The ratio of these areas describes the insulin output per unit secretory stimulus (insulinogenic index. The arrow marks the return of glucose to the fasting level. (b) Intravenous glucose tolerance tests in normal individuals and patients during burn resuscitation along with the insulin response. Data is described in Table 3.1.

that the 3—5 min Δ insulin level will adequately predict the physiologic responsiveness of the beta pancreatic cell.[6] Others have proposed that the 0—10 min insulinogenic index adequately quantifies the insulin response to a glucose load.

3.5   HOW IS THE FUNCTIONAL EFFECT OF INSULIN ON PERIPHERAL TISSUE DETERMINED? WHAT IS THE INSTANTANEOUS PROPORTIONALITY CONSTANT FOR GLUCOSE DISAPPEARANCE, OR *k*?

Insulin augments the translocation of glucose from the extracellular space to the intracellular compartment. The disappearance of glucose is determined following the rapid intravenous injection of a known glucose load or infusion of a constant glucose dose which is abruptly stopped (Fig. 3.3). Serial glucose determinations are obtained to quantitate the fall or disappearance of glucose from the glucose space (extracellular fluid compartment). The first approximation of the instantaneous proportionality constant for glucose disappearance (k, $100 \times min^{-1}$, or percent min^{-1}) is determined by plotting glucose concentration versus time on semilog graph paper and calculating the slope of the line,[7] but a more precise technique fits the data over a longer period of time until glucose concentration falls and achieves an equilibrium state (approaches an asymptotic level).[8] The constant k, multiplied by glucose concentration at any instant, determines the quantity of glucose disappearing from a volume of blood or serum at that instant. By calculating or estimating the "glucose space" (essentially the extracellular fluid compartment), the quantity of glucose disappearing from this compartment into the cells may be determined.

The constant k is elevated during exercise when muscle contraction facilitates entry of glucose into the cell and is normal or high normal in hyperthyroidism and during the hypermetabolic

[6]Lerner, R. L., and Porte, D., Jr.: Relationships between intravenous glucose loads, insulin response and glucose disappearance rate. *J. Clin. Endocr. Metab.*, 33:409, 1971.

[7]Samols, E., and Marks, V.: Interpretation of the intravenous glucose test. *Lancet,* 1:462, 1965.

[8]Hlad, C. J., Jr., Elrick, H., and Witten, T. A.: Studies on the kinetics of glucose utilization. *J. Clin. Invest.,* 35:1139, 1956.

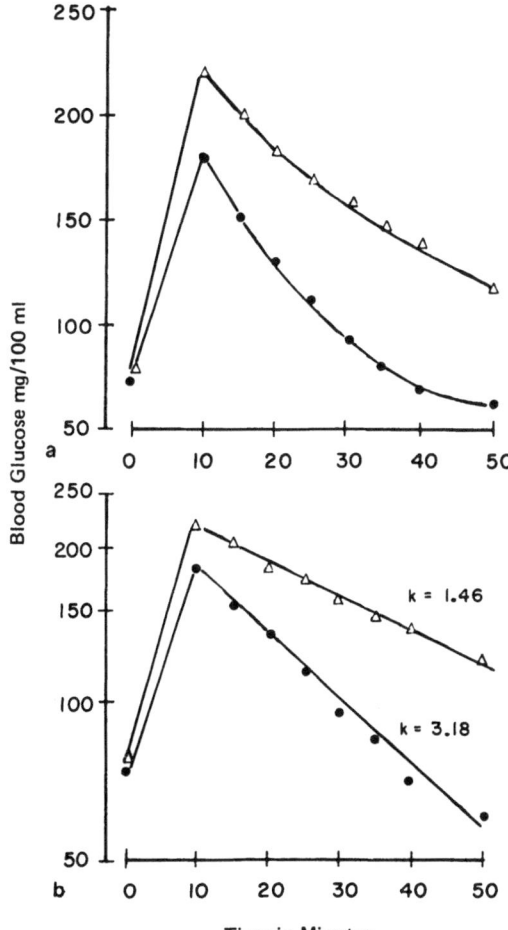

FIGURE 3.3: Following the intra-venous injection of 25 g glucose in normals and diabetic patients, serial blood samples for glucose are measured (a). The disappear-ance of glucose may be described by using a semilog plot (b) which linearizes the early portion of the disappearance curve. The slope of this line is k, or the instantaneous proportionality constant for glucose disappearance. • Normals, △ diabetics.

phase of thermal injury.[9] The k is decreased in diabetes, burn shock, hemorrhage, and during intracellular infection or bacteremia (Table 3.2). Because k reflects the influence of insulin on uptake of glucose in peripheral cells, the instantaneous proportionality constant for glucose disappearance is related to the quantity of insulin released following a glucose load and this association has been described in normals, diabetics, and injured patients (Fig. 3.4).

[9]Wilmore, D. W., Mason, A. D., Jr., and Pruitt, B. A., Jr.: Insulin response to glucose in hypermetabolic burn patients. *Ann. Surg.*, *183*:314, 1976.

Table 3.2   Effect of Stress on the Instantaneous
Proportionality Constant for Glucose
Disappearance

k decreased[a]	k normal or increased
Hypoxia	Exercise
Sepsis	Cold exposure
Bacterial	Hyperthyroidism
Viral	Burn hypermetabolism
Burn shock	
Hemorrhagic shock	
Myocardial infarction	
Anesthesia	
Operation	
Cerebral edema	

[a]Diabetic-like glucose tolerance curves.

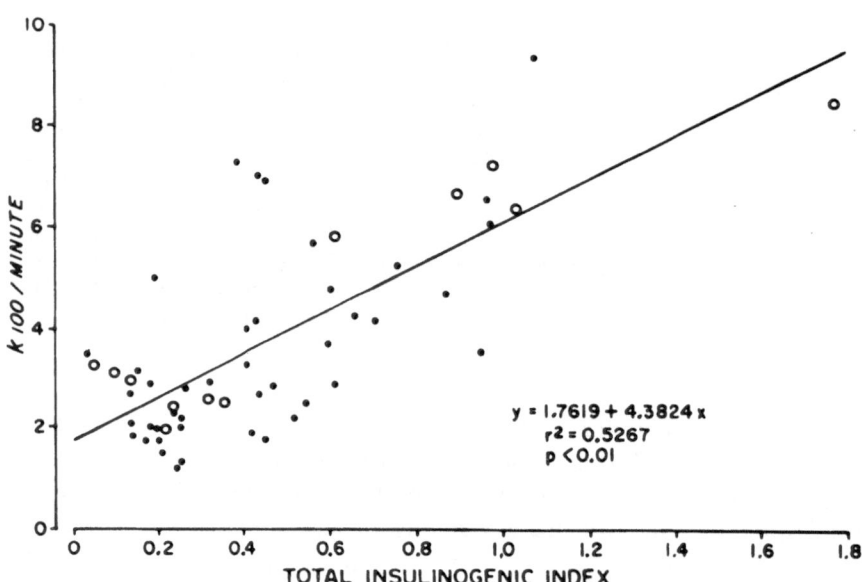

FIGURE 3.4: The central role of insulin in the peripheral disposal of glucose is demonstrated by the correlation between the instantaneous proportionality constant for glucose disappearance (k) and the insulin response (insulinogenic index). The greater the quantity of insulin released, the faster glucose disappears from the extracellular fluid compartment. A similar relationship is obtained in studies of patients with diabetes mellitus. ○ controls, ● burn patients.

Insulin augments transport of amino acids into peripheral tissue, and the branched-chain amino acids leucine, isoleucine, and valine pass through the liver and are largely degraded in skeletal muscle. Serum concentration of these amino acids reflects the insulin effect on peripheral tissue; branched-chain amino acid concentrations are elevated in the diabetic and decrease following insulin administration. In the patient with cirrhosis, insulin may bypass the liver because of the increased portal-systemic shunting which is present.[10] Peripheral tissue may become overinsulinized, which accounts for the low concentrations of branched-chain amino acids observed in patients with liver disease.

3.6   WHAT IS INSULIN'S EFFECT ON GLUCOSE METABOLISM?

Insulin is essential to glucose homeostasis: pancreatectomized man requires insulin for survival. Insulin responds to blood glucose to facilitate glucose entry into many tissues, increasing the flow of glucose along all pathways concerned with intracellular glucose metabolism. Thus, insulinized muscle increases formation of glycogen, lactic acid, and CO_2, and fat cells increase conversion of glucose to triglycerides in the presence of insulin. Glucose enters the liver and brain much more readily than muscle in the absence of insulin. In the liver, insulin induces key hepatic enzymes which favor storage of glycogen, suppresses hepatic enzymes concerned with glycolysis and gluconeogenesis, and reduces hepatic glucose production, an effect that is explained by the action of insulin on intracellular enzymes and is not dependent on increased hepatic membrane transport of glucose by insulin. Insulin lowers blood glucose by promoting removal of glucose by peripheral tissue and inhibiting hepatic glucose release; insulin also facilitates intracellular storage and/or metabolism of glucose.

3.7   HOW DOES INSULIN AFFECT FAT METABOLISM? . . . PROTEIN
METABOLISM?

Lipogenesis decreases in insulin-deprived man, and in the presence of lipolytic stimuli (such as catecholamines), the rate of triglyceride

---

[10]Munro, H. N., Fernstrom, J. D., and Wurtman, J. D.: Insulin, plasma amino acid imbalance, and hepatic coma. *Lancet, 1*:722, 1975.

breakdown is greatly accelerated when insulin concentrations are low. The mobilized free fatty acids may be converted in the liver to acetylacetate, acetone, or β-hydroxybutyrate, water-soluble compounds known as "ketone bodies." When serum insulin is low, such as in the glucose-deprived state, the rate of ketone production may exceed peripheral uptake, resulting in "ketosis"; significant quantities of ketones are found in blood and urine. Administration of carbohydrate and insulin reverses ketosis, promotes lipogenesis, and reduces the mobilization of free fatty acids and glycerol from the fat mass. The triglyceride stores are so sensitive to insulin that lypolysis will be inhibited by insulin alone in the absence of glucose. Insulin with dietary carbohydrate facilitates lipogenesis by aiding generation of acetyl—CoA from carbohydrate (a precursor of fatty acids), by providing alpha glycerol phosphate for esterification of fatty acids to form triglycerides, and by generation of NADPH, which is necessary for a key step in fat synthesis. The net result of the antilipolytic lipid synthetic glycerologenic actions of insulin is to convert energy ingested as carbohydrate to a storage form as lipid.

When the insulin concentration falls or insulin is absent, the efflux of amino acid from skeletal muscle increases. Insulinization of the skeletal muscle will reverse this effect by augmenting the transport of amino acids in the muscle cell[11] favoring protein synthesis. The increased amino acid transport, which occurs primarily in muscle, appears independent of the enhanced intracellular protein synthesis which is stimulated by insulin. In microsomes prepared from diabetic livers, amino acid incorporation is impaired and can be restored to normal by insulin.

Insulin is a critical hormone for the storage of carbohydrates and fat, and synthesis of new protein. It is a potent anabolic hormone which can counteract the negative nitrogen balance and catabolism of severe injury when administered with large quantities of glucose and potassium.[12]

[11]Pozefsky, T., Felig, P., and Tobin, J. D.: Amino acid balance across tissues of the forearm in postabsorptive man: Effects of insulin at two dose levels. *J. Clin. Invest. 48*:2273, 1969.

[12]Hinton, P., Allison, S. P., Littlejohn, S., and Lloyd, J.: Insulin and glucose to reduce catabolic response to injury in burn patients. *Lancet, 1*:767, 1971.

3.8   WHAT SUBSTANCES STIMULATE INSULIN RELEASE? WHAT HORMONES AFFECT INSULIN ELABORATION?

Insulin release occurs following glucose administration, and similar sugars exert comparable effects. The amount of insulin released is related quantitatively to the level of glucose in the blood. Nonmetabolized congeners of glucose (such as 2-deoxy-D-glucose) inhibit insulin secretion, suggesting that insulin release is regulated by the metabolism of glucose in the beta pancreatic cell. Insulin release is also stimulated by amino acids and products of lipid metabolism, long-chain free fatty acids and possibly ketone bodies. Thus, the three major fuels of the body influence the secretion of insulin.

It is well known that insulin response to an oral load of glucose is much greater than the response following a comparable intravenous dose of glucose. The differences in insulin responses have been attributed to hormonal factors in the upper duodenum (secretin and possibly pancreozymin), which act to prepare or sensitize the beta pancreatic cell to the intraluminal glucose. Other hormones affect insulin secretion, usually by altering insulin sensitivity to glucose, thus adjusting a response setpoint. For example, growth hormone increases the insulin response to a provocative stimulus (Fig. 3.5). Glucagon and ACTH directly stimulate insulin elaboration.

3.9   HOW DOES THE AUTONOMIC NERVOUS SYSTEM AFFECT THE ENDOCRINE PANCREAS?

The interaction between the autonomic nervous system and the endocrine pancreas is fundamental to the regulation of substrate storage or mobilization following stress. Catecholamines may suppress insulin release, and the increased sympathetic nervous system activity appears to be responsible for the insulin suppression and glucose intolerance observed during operation, volume depletion, mild or severe infection, and burn shock.[13] The insulin inhibitory effect of the sympathetic nervous system is mediated by alpha

---

[13]Porte, D., Jr., and Robertson, R. P.: Control of insulin secretion by catecholamines, stress, and the sympathetic nervous system. *Fed. Proc., 32*:1792, 1973.

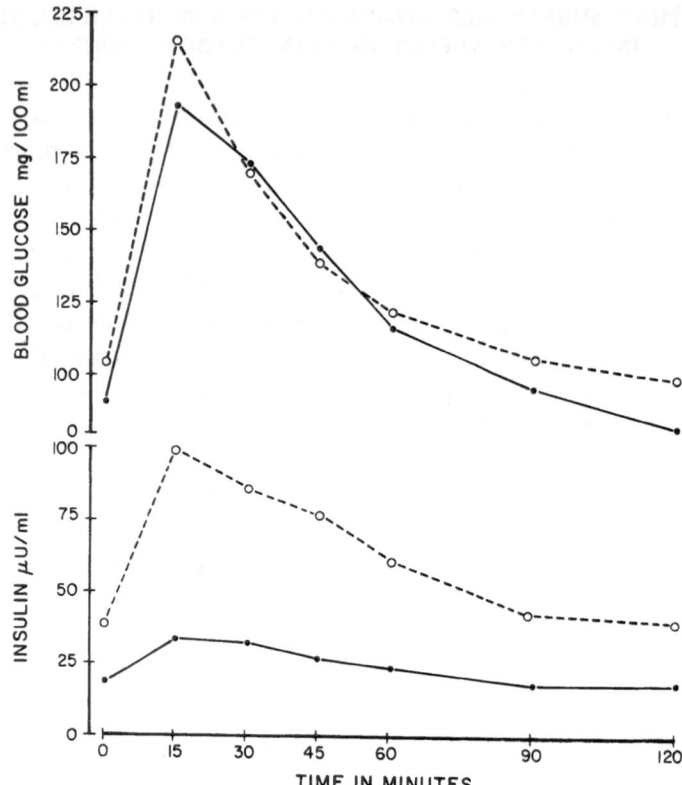

FIGURE 3.5: Mean glucose and insulin levels in six patients who received growth hormone, 10 IU daily for a week, during their posttraumatic catabolic course. Glucose tolerance curves obtained at the end of the week of therapy were compared with studies performed before hormone administration. Although dietary intake was constant throughout the study, a marked increase in the insulin response occurred with the HGH administration. •—• Control, o――o HGH.

receptors, while adrenergic beta receptor stimulation augments insulin elaboration.[14] During periods of marked sympathetic nervous system discharge, such as shock, myocardial infarction, or systemic infection, the alpha receptor effects appear to dominate, resulting in glucose intolerance. However, hypermetabolism, secondary to increased adrenergic activity, is characterized by increased heat production (a beta adrenergic effect), and increased mass flow of

[14]Iversen, J.: Adrenergic receptors and the secretion of glucagon and insulin from the isolated, perfused canine pancreas. *J. Clin. Invest., 52*:2102, 1973.

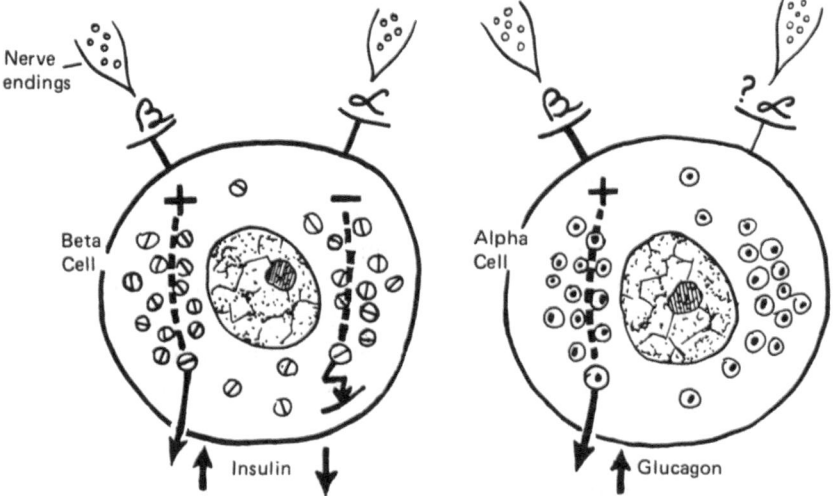

FIGURE 3.6: Insulin and glucagon release is stimulated by beta adrenergic receptors and insulin release is inhibited by alpha receptor stimulation. There is thought to be no alpha inhibitory effect on glucagon.

glucose from the liver to the peripheral tissue is related to the increased heat production which occurs. Beta adrenergic receptors may augment insulin elaboration during the "flow" phase of injury. Glucagon elaboration is stimulated by beta adrenergic receptors. The presence of an alpha inhibitory response on the alpha pancreatic cell has not been determined (Fig. 3.6).

3.10   WHAT ARE THE METABOLIC EFFECTS OF GLUCAGON? WHAT IS THE I/G RATIO?

Glucagon has potent glycolytic and gluconeogenic effects on the liver, hormonal properties precisely opposite those of insulin. Glucagon is proposed to be a hormone of "body glucose need," signaling the liver to make new glucose from hepatic glycogen stores or from gluconeogenic three-carbon precursors, providing additional glucose to the peripheral tissue. Unger and Orci have demonstrated that every hyperglycemic state except exogenous glucose administration is associated with hyperglucagonemia.[15] Maintenance of

[15]Unger, R. H., and Orci, L.: The essential role of glucagon in the pathogenesis of diabetes mellitus. *Lancet, 1*:14, 1975.

basal levels of blood glucose in normal man may be dependent on a
basal quantity of glucagon elaboration: suppression of basal glucagon
blood concentrations lowers fasting glucose levels significantly.[16] In
addition to its hyperglycemic effect, glucagon may augment ketosis,
a reaction which is abruptly stopped by insulin administration.

Unger has proposed that the insulin/glucagon (I/G) ratio be
utilized in a quantitative and qualitative sense to describe hepatic
glucose balance in fed and fasting man and diabetic patients.[17]
Anabolism and protein conservation occurs when insulin is increased
relative to glucagon (I/G > 5), a hormonal environment which favors
energy storage, limits gluconeogenesis, increases protein biosynthesis,
and decreases urea nitrogen excretion. Starvation in normal man,
diabetes, or infusion of glucagon into fasting man increase glucagon
relative to insulin (I/G < 3), and this hormonal milieu is associated
with increased glycogenolysis, gluconeogenesis, and ureagenesis at
the expense of protein biosynthesis.

3.11   WHAT STIMULATES GLUCAGON RELEASE?

Glucagon is stimulated by hypoglycemia, specific amino acids, other
three-carbon glucose intermediates, and the sympathetic nervous
system. Glucagon signals the liver to release glucose during states of
body glucose need, and hypoglycemia is a major signal for glucagon
release, which then stimulates hepatic glycogenolysis. Glucagon
partially regulates glucose homeostasis, and is stimulated by amino
acids, particularly the gluconeogenic amino acids that are converted
in the liver to new glucose. Amino acids also stimulate insulin
elaboration: essential amino acids have the greatest insulinogenic
potential (signaling for synthesis and storage of protein), while
nonessential amino acids have the most marked glucagon stimulating
effect (favoring conversion to glucose and/or transamination).
Alanine administration has been utilized as a provocative stimulus for
glucagon response measured in a variety of disease states. In addition

[16]Alford, F. P., Bloom, S. R., Nabarro, J. D. N., Hall, R., Besser, G. M., Coy, D. H., Kastin,
A. J., and Schally, A. V.: Glucagon control of fasting glucose in man. *Lancet,* 2:974,
1974.

[17]Unger, R. H.: Glucagon and the insulin:glucagon ratio in diabetes and other catabolic
illnesses. *Diabetes,* 20:834, 1971.

to amino acids, other three-carbon precursors, such as lactic acid, stimulate glucagon elaboration. As insulin monitors and normalizes blood glucose concentration in the extracellular compartment, glucagon senses alterations in the concentration of three-carbon fragments and acts to normalize these levels, primarily by converting these substances to glucose. Finally, glucagon elaboration is under the control of the autonomic nervous system and release is mediated by way of the beta adrenergic receptor system.

3.12 IS GLUCAGON THE HORMONE OF STRESS?

In traumatized or infected patients, glucagon levels are elevated even in the face of glucose administration and hyperglycemia.[18] The close relationship between glucagon and catecholamines in severely injured patients suggests that increased adrenergic activity may mediate the posttraumatic hyperglucagonemia which occurs after injury. The return of glucagon to normal coincides with healing of the wound when urine catecholamines fall to normal levels. Therefore, catecholamines appear to direct the pancreatic islet cell elaboration of both insulin and glucagon — that is, to adjust setpoints for the hormonal responses of the endocrine pancreas — and these hormones, in turn, control the disposition of key substrates under their control. Glucagon exerts its effect primarily on the liver, augmenting or amplifying catecholamine-directed, cyclic-AMP-mediated hepatic gluconeogenesis. Glucagon does not contribute to the efflux of amino acids from skeletal muscle.[19] Pancreatectomized patients can generate appropriate metabolic response to stress. Glucagon does not appear to be the primary stress hormone, but is permissive in its actions which appear to be primarily in the liver.

Glucagon rises during starvation, a response stimulated in part by the fall in blood glucose and an increase in plasma amino acids. The rise in glucagon and associated fall in insulin which occur in starved man appear to regulate hepatic glucose balance in this substrate deficient state.

[18]Wilmore, D. W., Lindsey, C. A., Moylan, J. A., Faloona, G. R., Pruitt, B. A., Jr., and Unger, R. H.: Hyperglucagonemia after burns. *Lancet*, 1:73, 1974.

[19]Fitzpatrick, G. F., Meguid, M. M., Gitlitz, P., O'Connor, N. E., and Brennan, M. F.: Effects of glucagon on 3-methylhistidine excretion: muscle proteolysis or ureogenesis? *Surg. Forum, 26*:46, 1975.

3.13   HOW ARE CATECHOLAMINES SYNTHESIZED, STORED, AND RELEASED?

Phenylalanine cannot be synthesized by the body and hence is an essential amino acid. Enzymatic conversion of phenylalanine to tyrosine occurs in the liver by a complex hydroxylation system, which is absent in children with phenylketonuria, and may be rate-limiting in patients with liver disease or premature infants with immature liver function. In man, it appears that the dietary source of tyrosine is the important precursor for synthesis of catecholamines.

Tyrosine is transported by the blood stream to various sites for catecholamine biosynthesis. It is transported across the cell membrane in specialized tissues by a tyrosine concentrating mechanism and undergoes a series of intracellular migrations — mitochondria, cytoplasm, storage vesicle — where specific enzymatic transformations occur, producing norepinephrine. The enzyme for conversion of norepinephrine to epinephrine is found in high concentrations in the adrenal medulla but not in the sympathetic nerve endings (Fig. 3.7).

The sympathetic neuron consists of a cell body, a long axon, and highly branched nerve terminals. The nerve terminals have swellings or varicosities which lie in close proximity to the effector cell, and it has been estimated that one neuron with its highly branched nerve endings may innervate some 25,000 effector cells.[20] Norepinephrine undergoes final biochemical processing and is stored as a nondiffusible complex of protein in the "granulated vesicles," which account for the varicosities of the nerve endings. With arrival of a nervous impulse, there is a change in ionic permeability of the membrane, permitting an influx of calcium. Although the effector mechanism is not known, norepinephrine and the other soluble compounds of the vesicle are discharged to the exterior of the nerve terminal. The released norepinephrine diffuses across the synaptic cleft between the nerve ending and the effector cell, where it interacts with specific adrenergic receptors.[21]

Epinephrine is stored in the adrenal medulla and is released by sympathetic nerve stimulation. Epinephrine exerts its effects on

---

[20]Wurtman, R. J.: Catecholamines. *New Eng. J. Med.,* 273: 637, 1965.
[21]Axelrod, J., and Weinshilboum, R.: Catecholamines. *New Eng. J. Med.,* 287:237, 1972.

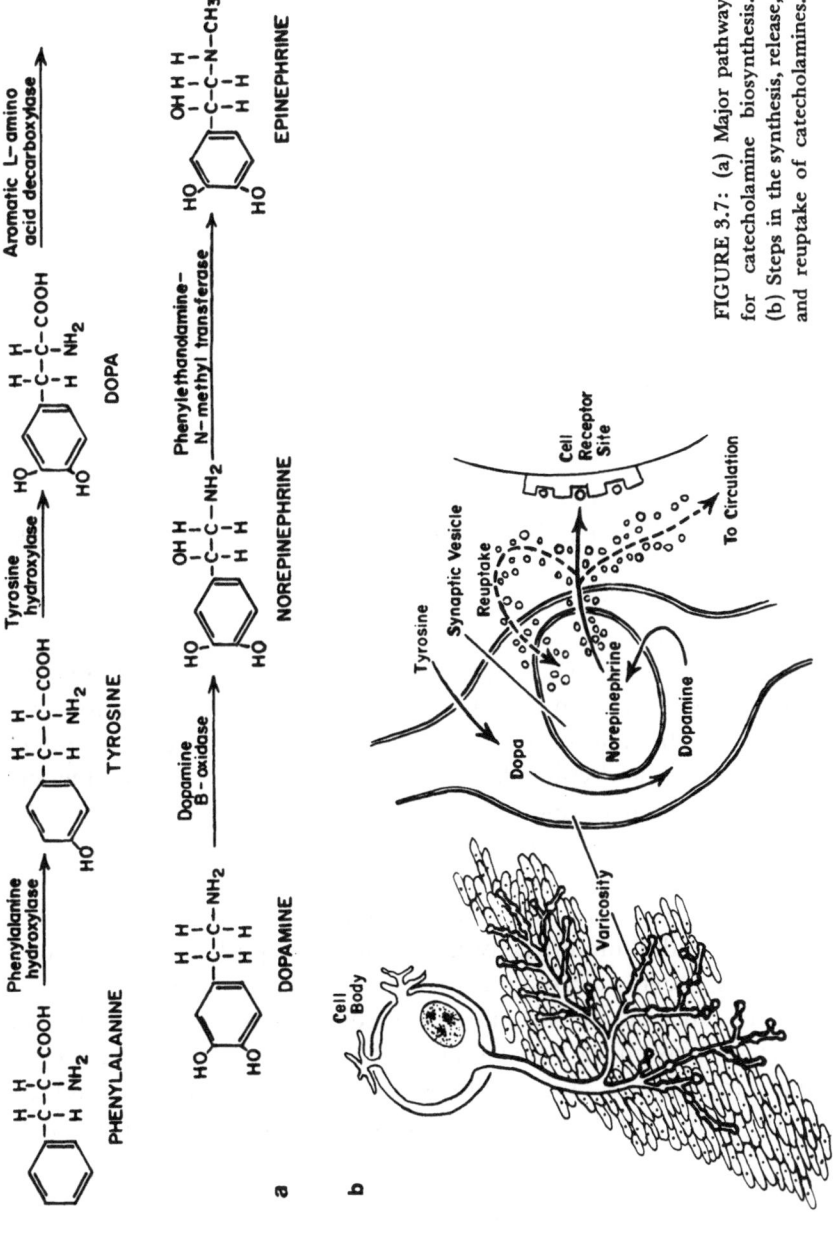

FIGURE 3.7: (a) Major pathway for catecholamine biosynthesis. (b) Steps in the synthesis, release, and reuptake of catecholamines.

distant target organs and, unlike norepinephrine, is carried to effector cells by the blood stream. Dopamine is a specific intermediate compound for the synthesis of epinephrine and norepinephrine, but it also stimulates specific receptors in the central nervous system and may act as a transmitter in the peripheral autonomic nervous system.

3.14   HOW IS CATECHOLAMINE ACTIVITY ASSESSED?

The major portion of released norepinephrine is taken up again and stored in the sympathetic nerve ending. Only a small fraction of the released norepinephrine escapes this recapture mechanism and diffuses into the blood stream to appear in plasma or urine.

Catecholamines do not diffuse from the central nervous system to contribute to blood or urine levels. Adrenal medullary output is directly reflected by blood and urinary catecholamine concentrations.

The generally accepted method for determining quantitative sympathetic nervous system activity in man is to measure catecholamine excretion rate in the urine.[22] This limits the measurements to individuals with normal renal function and circulation. In addition to measuring the free catecholamines, norepinephrine and epinephrine, their breakdown products (metanephrine, normetanephrine, VMA, etc.) that are excreted in the urine can be quantitated. Concentration of catecholamines can be measured in the blood, but the usual fluorometric technique requires a large serum volume. More recently, measurements of serum catecholamines by radioimmunoassay has been accomplished, and this technique may provide a rapid sensitive serum analysis in time.

Serum analysis of the one intermediate enzyme, dopamine-β-hydroxylase, may index catecholamine turnover.[23] This enzyme is not subject to reuptake and readily enters the blood stream after release. Its circulating half-life is considerably longer than that of norepine-

[22]Von Euler, U. S.: Quantitation of stress by catecholamine analysis. *Clin. Pharm. Therap.*, *5*:398, 1964.
[23]Geffen, L.: Serum dopamine β-hydroxylase as an index of sympathetic function. *Life Sci.*, *14*:1593, 1974.

phrine. Measurement of serum concentrations of this enzyme may be a useful indicator of sympathetic activity and turnover of epinephrine and norepinephrine stores.

It should be reemphasized that norepinephrine, which is the major hormone of the sympathetic nervous system, transmits messages to effector cells from nerve endings which are in intimate contact with the target organ. Anatomic studies confirm the presence of a rich plexus of sympathetic and parasympathetic nerve endings in metabolic target organs such as the liver and pancreas. The major portion of norepinephrine produced in these nerve endings is either recaptured by the same nerves or degraded by effector cells, and blood and/or urine measurements only roughly quantitate actual sympathetic activity. A variety of physiological techniques have been utilized to measure sympathetic activity and the responses of the autonomic nervous system to stress. The cold-pressor test is an example of a test technique which evaluates a sympathetic reflex response. Cold exposure and pyrogen administration are additional methods utilized to stimulate the sympathetic nervous system and assess its response. The response to infused catecholamine – the delivery of norepinephrine to the effector cells by the blood stream rather than by direct nerve stimulation and diffusion through the synaptic cleft – should be equated to the physiologic response only if similar effects are obtained following stimulation of the intact sympathetic nervous system (utilizing cold exposure or pyrogen administration).

Investigative techniques exist to assess the size of the active catecholamine pool (tyramine stimulation, cold response) and determine turnover of the various precursors of catecholamine.[24] Sympathetic tissue and target organs have been assayed to determine the quantity of catecholamine stores in nerve vesicles, sympathetic ganglion, adrenal medulla, and myocardium. These studies all confirm that depletion of the catecholamine stores occurs in patients with prolonged illness. Finally, sympathetic activity may be blocked by specific pharmacologic agents to aid assessment of the sympathetic nervous system in response to a specific disease process.

[24]Goodall, McC., and Alton, H.: Dopamine (3-hydroxytyramine) replacement and metabolism in sympathetic nerve and adrenal medullary depletions after prolonged thermal injury. J. Clin. Invest., 48:1761, 1969.

3.15   WHY ARE CATECHOLAMINES CALLED THE HORMONES OF STRESS?

Walter B. Cannon and his colleagues provided convincing evidence that the catecholamines were liberated during stress, and were in fact essential for maintaining body homeostasis following a wide variety of stressful stimuli.[25] Utilizing the rate of the denervated heart as a biological indicator of adrenal medullary catecholamine release, Cannon found heart rate increased with fright, rage, pain, asphyxia, anesthesia, muscular activity, cold exposure, and sensory nerve stimulation. Removal or denervation of the adrenal glands, or ligation of the adrenal veins, abolished this response. He then removed all of the sympathetic ganglion from cats; the animals remained in good health, lived long lives, and the females even reproduced as long as they were maintained in the sheltered environment of the laboratory. However, the sympathectomized animals were particularly vulnerable to stress, and unable to defend against hypoxia, fluid restriction, variations in environmental temperature, hemorrhage, and exercise. The sympathetic nervous system, transmitting signals by way of the catecholamines, was *essential for survival during stress.*

3.16   WHAT ARE THE GENERAL EFFECTS OF SUDDEN SYMPATHETIC NERVOUS SYSTEM DISCHARGE? WHAT ARE THE EFFECTS OF EPINEPHRINE AND NOREPINEPHRINE INFUSION IN MAN?

The dramatic effect of sudden sympatho-adrenal discharge is observed in an injured animal. The "fight-or-flight" syndrome is characterized by tachycardia, pupillary dilatation, pilo-erector activity of the skin, alterations in skin and muscle blood flow, and an increased respiratory rate associated with bronchial dilatation. This physiologic response is accompanied by an outpouring of glucose and free fatty acids into the blood stream and release of hormones which signal for salt and water retention. Cuthbertson has emphasized that at the time of injury there may be a depression in the physiologic response to the hormonal discharge ("ebb phase"), which may be transitory and a manifestation of circulatory inadequacy or

[25]Cannon, W. B.: *The Wisdom of the Body.* New York, Norton, pp. 177–201, 1967.

neurogenic shock. If the organism survives the initial injury, the early response is generally followed by an increase in metabolic reactions ("flow phase"), presumably to provide substrate for the inflammatory response and tissue repair.

The characteristic effects of hormonal infusion in man are shown in Table 3.3.

Table 3.3   Comparison of the Effects of Intravenous
Infusion of Epinephrine and Norepinephrine in Man

	Epinephrine[a]	Norepinephrine[a]
Cardiac		
Heart rate	+	−
Stroke volume	++	++
Cardiac output	+++	0, −
Arrhythmias	++++	++++
Coronary blood flow	++	++
Blood pressure		
Systolic arterial	+++	+++
Mean arterial	+	++
Diastolic arterial	+, 0, −	++
Mean pulmonary	++	++
Peripheral circulation		
Total peripheral resistance	−	++
Cerebral blood flow	+	0, −
Muscle blood flow	+++	0, −
Cutaneous blood flow	− −	− −
Renal blood flow	−	−
Splanchnic blood flow	+++	0, +
Metabolic effects		
Oxygen consumption	++	0, +
Blood sugar	+++	0, +
Blood lactic acid	+++	0, +
Eosinopenic response	+	0
Central nervous system		
Respiration	+	+
Subjective sensations	+	+

[a]+ = Increase, 0 = No change, − = Decrease.
Adapted from: Goodman, L. S., and Gilman, A., *The Pharmacological Basis of Therapeutics*, 5th Ed., New York, MacMillan, 1975, p. 485.

3.17 WHAT ARE ALPHA AND BETA RECEPTORS? HOW ARE THEY DETERMINED? WHAT DO THEY DO?

Catecholamines elicit a variety of physiologic effects: specific tissues may respond in an opposite manner when the effect of epinephrine is compared to the norepinephrine response. In addition, a low dose of neurohormone may elicit an entirely different response than the high dose of catecholamine. These paradoxical effects are attributed to the presence of a dual receptor system present in most tissues. With utilization of pharmacologic blocking agents, a specific effect can be attenuated by competitive receptor blockade, and the response attributed to alpha- or beta-adrenergic receptor stimulation, depending upon the blocking agent used (Table 3.4). Epinephrine

Table 3.4   Responses of Effector Organs to Autonomic Nerve Impulses

Effector organs	Adrenergic impulses[a]		Cholinergic impulses[b]
	Receptor type	Responses[c]	Responses[c]
Heart			
S-A nodes	β	Increase in heart rate++	Decrease in heart rate; vagal arrest+++
Atria	β	Increase in contractility and conduction velocity++	Decrease in contractility and (usually) increase in conduction velocity++
A-V node	β	Increase in automaticity and conduction velocity++	Decrease in conduction velocity; A-V block+++
His-Purkinje system	β	Increase in automaticity and conduction velocity+++	Little effect
Ventricles	β	Increase in contractility, conduction velocity, automaticity, and rate of idioventricular pacemakers+++	Slight decrease in contractility claimed by some
Arterioles			
Coronary	α β	Constriction+; dilatation++	Dilatation±
Skin and mucosa	α	Constriction+++	Dilatation
Skeletal muscle	α β	Constriction++; dilatation++	Dilatation+
Cerebral	α	Constriction (slight)	Dilatation
Pulmonary	α β	Constriction+; dilatation	Dilatation
Abdominal viscera; renal	α β	Constriction+++; dilatation+	———

Continued

Table 3.4—continued

| Effector organs | Adrenergic impulses[a] | | Cholinergic impulses[b] |
	Receptor type	Responses[c]	Responses[c]
Salivary glands	α	Constriction+++	Dilatation++
Veins (systemic)	α	Constriction++	————
Lung			
Bronchial muscle	β	Relaxation+	Contraction++
Bronchial glands		Inhibition (?)	Stimulation+++
Stomach			
Motility and tone	β	Decrease (usually)+	Increase+++
Sphincters	α	Contraction (usually)+	Relaxation (usually)+
Secretion		Inhibition (?)	Stimulation+++
Intestine			
Motility and tone	α β	Decrease+	Increase+++
Sphincters	α	Contraction (usually)+	Relaxation (usually)+
Secretion		Inhibition (?)	Stimulation++
Gallbladder and ducts		Relaxation+	Contraction+
Urinary bladder			
Detrusor	β	Relaxation (usually)+	Contraction+++
Trigone and sphincter	α	Contraction++	Relaxation++
Skin			
Pilomotor muscles	α	Contraction++	————
Sweat glands	α	Localized secretion+	Generalized secretion+++
Spleen capsule	α β	Contraction+++; relaxation+	————
Adrenal medulla		————	Secretion of epinephrine and norepinephrine
Liver	β	Glycogenolysis, gluconeogenesis, etc.+++	Glycogen synthesis+
Pancreas			
Acini	α	Decreased secretion+	Secretion++
Islet (B cells)	α	Decreased secretion+++	————
	β	Increased secretion+	————
Fat cells	β	Lipolysis+++	————
Salivary glands	α	Potassium and water· secretion+	Potassium and water secretion+++
	β	Amylase secretion+++	————

[a] From neurons which release norepinephrine.
[b] From neurons which release acetylcholine.
[c] Responses range from +1 to +3.
Adapted from: Goodman, L. S., and Gilman, A.: *The Pharmacological Basis of Thera-peutics*, 5th Ed., Macmillan, New York, 1975, pp. 408–409.

and norepinephrine exhibit stimulatory properties of both receptor systems, but epinephrine exerts predominantly beta effects and norepinephrine exhibits predominantly alpha characteristics. With the characterization of cyclic AMP, the second or "intracellular" messenger, the adrenergic beta receptor system has been proposed as an integral part of the adenyl cyclase system.[26] Beta receptor stimulation causes an increase in the intracellular level of cyclic AMP. Conversely, alpha receptor effects might be mediated by a fall in the intracellular concentrations of cyclic AMP.

3.18   HOW DO CATECHOLAMINES STIMULATE HYPERGLYCEMIA?

Hyperglycemia occurs following the injection of epinephrine as a response to a complex series of interactions. First, there is a direct effect on the liver, increasing the conversion rate of glycogen to glucose and simultaneously directing conversion of three-carbon precursors to glucose. Second, epinephrine acts directly on skeletal muscle, converting skeletal muscle glycogen to lactic acid which is transported to the liver and converted to new glucose (Cori cycle). Beta receptors characteristically mediate this effect. Finally, epinephrine has a direct effect on the pancreas, suppressing the release of insulin that would normally occur in response to an elevated blood glucose level. Simultaneously, pancreatic glucagon is stimulated, augmenting the signal for hepatic glucose release.

3.19   HOW DO CATECHOLAMINES AFFECT FAT MOBILIZATION?

Mobilization of free fatty acids occurs following sympathetic stimulation, a result of the direct action of catecholamines on fat cells. This effect is blocked by adrenergic blocking agents and nicotinic acid. The lipolytic effect of catechols is potentiated by suppression of insulin release from the pancreatic beta cell; low insulin levels favor fat mobilization, while high insulin concentrations augment fat storage. Glucose administration to critically ill patients

[26]Robinson, G. A., Butcher, R. W., and Sutherland, E. W.: *Cyclic AMP.* New York, Academic Press, 1971, p. 145.

will stimulate endogenous insulin, limit fat mobilization, and allow oxidation of the infused carbohydrate. Thus, fat mobilization is regulated by an interaction of insulin and catecholamines, with insulin favoring fat storage and sympathetic activity stimulating mobilization.

3.20   DO CATECHOLAMINES STIMULATE HEAT PRODUCTION?

The calorigenic effects of catecholamines may represent one of the most important effects of these hormones. Catecholamines infused into animals increase metabolic rate, and epinephrine or norepinephrine infusions in normal man produce hypermetabolism. Rats in which adrenergic function is completely blocked die in 3 hr when exposed to 4°C ambient environment, while normal animals adjust to the temperature by increasing their metabolic rate.[27] These effects are blocked by beta-adrenergic receptor antagonist but are not affected by alpha blockade.

Recent experiments on the cellular mechanisms of thermogenesis suggest that specialized tissues (brown fat) respond to catecholamine stimulation by increasing sodium pump activity, which in turn, increases cellular heat production.[28]

3.21   WHAT STIMULATES HEAT PRODUCTION IN THE CRITICALLY ILL PATIENT?

Present evidence indicates that hypermetabolism in hospitalized patients is the result of increased sympathetic outflow. Catecholamines are elevated following thermal injury and infection, and adrenergic activity has been related to the extent of injury and to the oxygen consumption of the patient. Carefully controlled adrenergic blockade in patients with large surface area burns demonstrated a consistent decrease in metabolic rate with alpha- and beta- or beta-adrenergic blockade alone. Administration of epinephrine and

[27]Brodie, B. B., Davies, J. I., Hynie, S., Krishna, G., and Weiss, B.: Interrelationships of catecholamines with other endocrine systems. *Pharm. Rev., 18*:273, 1966.
[28]Horwitz, B. A.: Ouabain-sensitive component of brown fat thermogenesis. *Amer. J. Physiol, 224*:352, 1973.

norepinephrine to normal man increases metabolic activity (Fig. 3.8). Increased catecholamines (increased adrenergic activity) are the major calorigenic mediators responsible for the posttraumatic hypermetabolic response following injury. Increased calorigenesis has also been noted with growth hormone administration and infusion of glucagon, both hormones which are elevated in injured man. The physiologic significance of these effects is yet to be determined, but these hormonal mediators may augment or potentiate the catecholamine-directed heat production which occurs in injured man.

Infection causes a reset in the temperature center of the hypothalamus. Hypothalamic centers then act to increase sympathetic activity and elevate body temperature by (1) causing

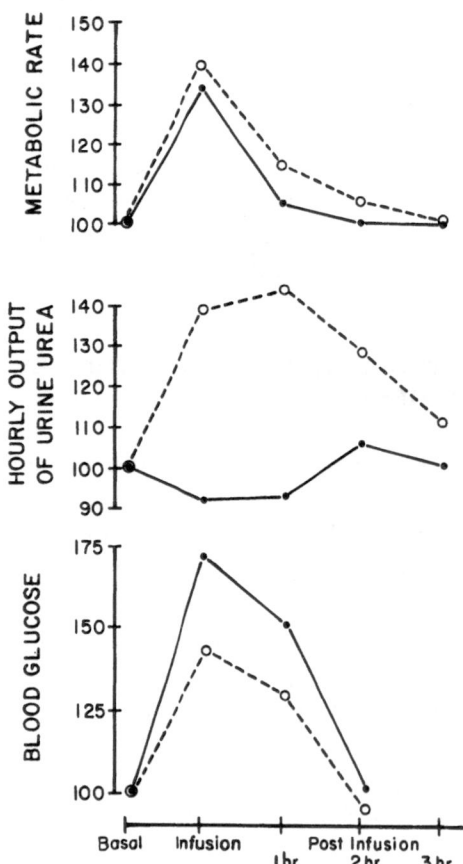

FIGURE 3.8: The metabolic response of fed and fasting men to an infusion of epinephrine, 6 μg/min. Hypermetabolism and hyperglycemia occur in both groups, but, in the fasted subjects with depleted glycogen stores, increased excretion of urinary nitrogen also occurs. ●—● Fed $n = 5$, o———o Fasting $n = 6$.

vasoconstriction which decreases heat loss, and/or (2) stimulating hypermetabolism which increases heat production. Temperature reset appears to occur in injured man although the afferent stimulus for this response is poorly understood.

3.22   WHAT LIMITS THE BODY'S RESPONSE TO CATECHOLAMINE-MEDIATED STIMULI?

The ability to respond to a stimulus requiring catecholamine calorigenesis depends upon the availability of catecholamine reserves and the ability of tissues to respond to increased catechol stimuli. Studies evaluating catecholamine stores in patients who die following injury and stress demonstrate depletion of these neurotransmitter reserves in the adrenal medulla, sympathetic nerve endings and sympathetic ganglion, and the heart. Dopamine turnover in burn patients is markedly increased and serum tyrosine concentrations may be altered, possibly reflecting substrate limitation. Burn patients with injuries of more than 40% of the body surface appear to maintain maximal or near-maximal rates of catecholamine synthesis and utilization. Exposing these patients to a cool environment (21°C) results in a mild cold stress, ordinarily a stimulus for the elaboration of additional catecholamines. Patients who eventually survived responded by increasing heat production as a result of elaboration of catecholamines. In contrast, patients who lacked catecholamine reserves or tissue responsiveness to these mediators failed to generate additional heat to maintain heat balance in the 21°C ambient temperature and became hypothermic (Fig. 3.9). All of the nonresponding patients subsequently died from complications of their injuries. Like Cannon's sympathectomized cats, the non-responders lacked homeostatic reserve, for injury had reset their rates of energy production at a maximal level. Additional sympathetic nervous system reserves were unavailable for catecholamine-mediated responses to cooling, infection, and hemorrhage.

3.23   WHAT STIMULATES ACTH? WHAT IS THE FUNCTION OF ACTH?

Early work with hypophysectomized animals demonstrated the dependence of the adrenal cortex on pituitary activity, and the

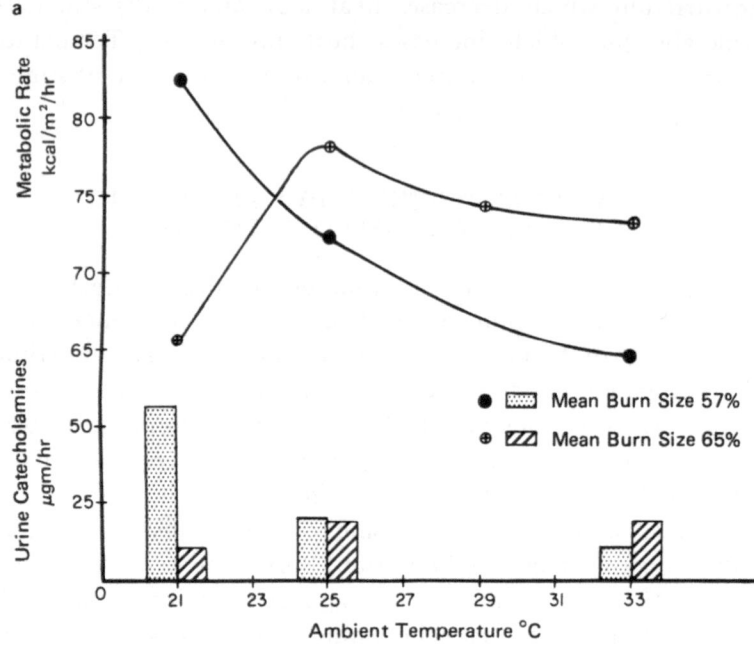

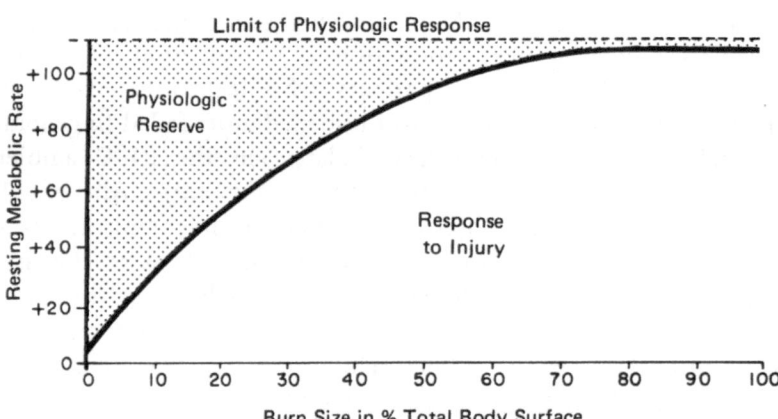

FIGURE 3.9: (a) The inability of patients with large thermal injury to respond to a mild cold stress suggests that these individuals are at maximal rates of energy production and cannot respond appropriately to additional catechol-mediated stress, such as cooling, infection, and hemorrhage. (b) Physiological reserve decreases as the extent of injury or infection increases.

transmitting hormone was later found to be the polypeptide ACTH (adrenocorticotropin). The hypothalamic centers which stimulate ACTH secretion are under three general types of control. First, ACTH levels fluctuate throughout the day, peak just before awakening in the morning, and are low during the early hours of sleep. This rhythm is determined by higher centers in the brain. Secondly, corticosteroid levels in the plasma exert a depressing effect on corticotropin-releasing factor (the hypothalamic factor which stimulates ACTH synthesis and pituitary release). Increased steroid levels reduce ACTH in the blood and pituitary gland. Finally, a wide variety of stresses, both psychological and physical, stimulate ACTH release.

In a series of classic studies, Hume and Egdahl measured adrenal venous 17-hydroxycorticosteroids in experimental animals and demonstrated that the adrenocorticoid secretion was not elicited after trauma to a denervated hind limb.[29] The adrenocortical response to injury was not observed after transection of the peripheral nerve to the area of the trauma, transection of the spinal cord above the injury, or section through the medulla oblongata. Other studies demonstrated that the posttraumatic elevation of ACTH and adrenocorticoids could be abolished in animals subjected to standard operative trauma with previously placed electrical lesions in the anterior medial eminence or following hypophysectomy. Removing the cortex of the brain or sectioning the pituitary stalk did not ablate the ACTH response to injury. Blunting the ACTH responses by denervation of the extremity before operation has also been described in man. ACTH elaboration appears to be the major stimulus for corticosteroid elaboration, and there appears to be no direct nervous control of adrenal cortical activity. Denervation of the gland does not alter adrenal cortical function.

ACTH stimulates secretion of cortisol and corticosterone, but not aldosterone. The extraadrenal effects of ACTH include the ability to release free fatty acids, promote insulin secretion, and reduce deamination of amino acids. ACTH reduces the concentration of ascorbic acid in the adrenal gland. Although the interaction

[29]Hume, D. M., and Egdahl, R. H.: The importance of the brain in the endocrine response to injury. *Ann. Surg., 150*:697, 1959.

between ascorbic acid and adrenal secretion is not well understood, assay of adrenal ascorbic acid level is a useful method for ACTH assay in animals.

3.24   HOW IS CORTISOL TRANSPORTED IN THE BLOOD?

The cortisol and other corticosteroids elaborated by the adrenal gland into the plasma may be bound to a specific corticosteroid-binding globulin, bound to albumin, or circulate as the free active form. The bound hormone cannot actively penetrate membranes and is metabolically inactive, but the bound hormone maintains an equilibrium with the free steroid and thus acts as a reservoir as free steroid is removed from the plasma. Most assays of the hormone in the blood determine free cortisone.

3.25   HOW ARE THE CORTICOSTEROIDS CLASSIFIED?

The effects of steroids can be classified into two general categories: (1) those concerned with organic metabolism (metabolism of fat, carbohydrate, and protein; inflammation; wound healing; and myocardial metabolism), and (2) those affecting mineral metabolism.

Steroids are classified in terms of their relative glucocorticoid and mineralocorticoid activity, and the hormones have been arranged in increasing ratios of glucocorticoid to mineralocorticoid activities.

Commercially available glucocorticoid compounds may be classified as short-, intermediate-, and long-acting on the basis of their ACTH suppression (Table 3.5).

3.26   WHAT ARE THE PRIMARY EFFECTS OF GLUCOCORTICOIDS ON METABOLISM?

1. *Promote Gluconeogenesis*. Glucocorticoids provide specific signals to augment hepatic gluconeogenesis by stimulating enzymes which direct conversion of three-carbon fragments into synthesis of new glucose. Glucocorticoids augment other hormonal signals for the production of new glucose and increased gluconeogenesis

Table 3.5   Commonly Used Glucocorticoids

Duration of action	Glucocorticoid patency (relative)	Equivalent glucocorticoid dose (mg)	Mineralocorticoid activity
Short-acting			
Cortisol (hydrocortisone)	1	20	yes[a]
Cortisone	0.8	25	yes[a]
Prednisone	4	5	no
Prednisolone	4	5	no
Methylprednisolone	5	4	no
Intermediate-acting			
Triamcinolone	5	4	no
Long-acting			
Betamethasone	25	0.60	no
Dexamethasone	30	0.75	no

[a]Mineralocorticoid effects are dose-related. At doses close to or within the basal physiologic range for glucocorticoid activity no such effect may be detectable.
Adapted from: Axelrod, L.: Glucocorticoid therapy, *Medicine, 55*:42, 1976.

occurs in animals when corticosteroids are administered in conjunction with catecholamines. In addition, glucocorticoids promote storage of carbohydrate as glycogen. Adrenalectomized animals demonstrate reduction of urinary nitrogen, blood glucose, and liver glycogen, and these concentrations are restored to normal with steroid administration.

2. *Mobilize Amino Acids.* The stable adrenalectomized animal cannot mobilize amino acids from skeletal muscle. However, there is no impairment in utilization of free amino acids provided in the diet or by intravenous administration. As long as the animal is fed, it can maintain carbohydrate stores and continue protein biosynthesis; when forced to depend on its own protein stores for carbohydrate precursors or for hepatic protein synthesis, the adrenalectomized animal cannot meet this demand. This effect is reversed by glucocorticoid administration. Although glucocorticoids facilitate amino acid mobilization from the periphery, protein biosynthesis is favored in the liver, resulting in the overall movement of protein from the carcass to the viscera.

3. *Alter Fat Metabolism.* Although the precise effect of cortisol is not completely clear, steroids increase body fat. Adrenal insuf-

ficiency is associated with decreased triglyceride and cholesterol synthesis in humans. Glucocorticoids augment lipolysis and catecholamine-stimulated glycogen oxidation in skeletal muscle. The overall effect on body composition following glucocorticoid administration is the erosion of lean body mass while body fat is maintained or increased. Extracellular water is also increased.

The Effect of Glucocorticoids on Carbohydrate and Protein Metabolism

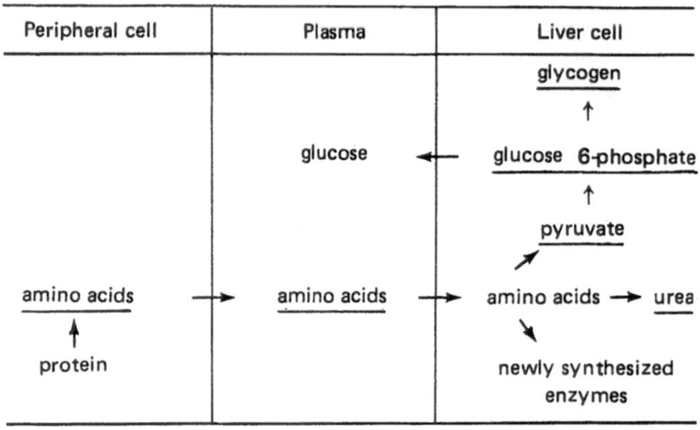

Peripheral cell	Plasma	Liver cell
		glycogen
		↑
	glucose ⟵	glucose 6-phosphate
		↑
		pyruvate
		↗
amino acids ⟶	amino acids ⟶	amino acids ⟶ urea
↑		↘
protein		newly synthesized enzymes

FIGURE 3.10: The substances underlined are increased in concentration with steroid administration and the heavy arrows indicate the pathways of flow. Adapted from Bondy, P. K.: The adrenal cortex. *Diseases of Metabolism*. Philadelphia, W. B. Saunders, 1969, p. 845.

3.27   ARE GLUCOCORTICOIDS THE HORMONES RESPONSIBLE FOR NEGATIVE NITROGEN BALANCE FOLLOWING INJURY?

Blood levels of steroids increase following injury or stress. Because of the amino acid mobilizing and gluconeogenic properties, corticosteroids were once thought to be responsible for the posttraumatic metabolic changes. However, adrenalectomized animals maintained on a constant dose of glucocorticoids respond to injury in the expected manner.[30] Thus, the effect of glucocorticoids was defined as permissive, augmenting or amplifying specific metabolic responses to stress but not the primary cause of the response. Glucocorticoids

[30]Ingle, D. J., Meeks, R. C., and Thomas, K. E.: The effect of fractures upon urinary electrolytes in non-adrenalectomized rats and in adrenalectomized rats treated with adrenal cortex extract. *Endocrinology*, 49:703, 1951.

administered to fasting man do not increase nitrogen excretion,[31] and the protein wasting associated with systemic infection is not attributed to the effects of endogenous corticosteroids.[32]

3.28 DO THE ANTIINFLAMMATORY EFFECTS OF CORTICOSTEROIDS INFLUENCE THE BODY'S SYSTEMIC RESPONSE TO INFECTION OR INJURY?

When the body's inflammatory response is elicited by infection, a physical agent, or foreign body, the administration of corticosteroids prevents the full expression of the inflammatory response. Steroids prevent full dilation of capillaries; cellular exudate is reduced, transudation and edema are diminished, less fibrin is deposited in the inflamed area, and healing is delayed. Steroids also cause a rapid destruction of lymphocytes and a reduction of the antibody response. These factors intimately involved in the inflammatory response may liberate humoral factors ("endogenous pyrogen," histamine, prostaglandins) that may evoke or effect a systemic metabolic response. Alteration of the normal inflammatory response could affect the host's ability to mount a systemic response to the local inflammatory process.

3.29 DOES INCREASED GROWTH HORMONE ELABORATION OCCUR FOLLOWING STRESS?

Yes. Growth hormone elaboration occurs following a wide variety of stressful situations including hypoglycemia, exercise, hemorrhage, operation, thermal injury, infection, and starvation. Some stimuli which promote growth hormone elaboration may be suppressed by hyperglycemia while others augment growth hormone elaboration in spite of the elevation of blood glucose (Table 3.6).

   Amino acids are potent stimulating agents and arginine infusion has been utilized to test the pituitary capacity to release growth

---

[31]Owens, O. E., and Cahill, G. F., Jr.: Metabolic effects of exogenous glucocorticoids in fasting man. *J. Clin. Invest.*, *52*:2596, 1973.

[32]Beisel, W. R., Sawyer, W. D., Ryll, E. D., and Crozier, D.: Metabolic effects of intracellular infections in man. *Ann. Int. Med.*, *67*:744, 1967.

Table 3.6   Normal Stimuli for Growth Hormone Secretion

Suppressed by glucose	Independent of glucose
Basal resting	Pyrogen
Hypoglycemia	Major operations
Rapid fall in blood glucose without hypoglycemia	Intravenous amino acids
Inhibition of intracellular glucose utilization	L-Dopa administration
Prolonged fasting	
Muscular exercise	

Adapted from: Roth, J. (moderator), Glick, S. M., Cuatrecasas, P., and Hollander, C.: Acromegaly and other disorders of growth hormone secretion, presented at the Combined Clinical Staff Conference of the National Institutes of Health. *Ann. Int. Med., 66:*760, 1967, and Martin, J. B.: Neural regulation of growth hormone secretion. *New Eng. J. Med., 288:*1384, 1973.

hormone. Insulin hypoglycemia is a strong provocative stimulus utilized to assess growth hormone elaboration. Growth hormone is elevated following injury in spite of persistent hyperglycemia which would suppress growth hormone elaboration in normal man. Moreover, the hormonal response to both insulin hypoglycemia and arginine infusion is decreased in injured man, demonstrating further alterations in hypothalamic control which may occur following stress (Fig. 3.11). Morphine anesthesia will diminish or abolish the increase in growth hormone which occurs during operation.

3.30   WHAT ARE THE ACTIONS OF GROWTH HORMONE?

This single-chain polypeptide stimulates nucleic acid and protein synthesis in a wide variety of tissues and stimulates synthesis of chondroitin sulfate and collagen. The dramatic effect of this highly potent anabolic hormone is demonstrated with growth hormone administration to an immature, deficient organism: prompt linear growth and weight gain result. Growth hormone promotes protein storage, increases fat mobilization and utilization, and resets the insulin response to glucose. These and other actions of growth hormone are shown in Table 3.7.

3.31   CAN THE ANABOLIC EFFECTS OF GROWTH HORMONE REVERSE THE CATABOLIC EFFECTS OF INJURY AND INFECTION?

Yes, human growth hormone administration, with sufficient calories and protein to maintain energy and nitrogen balance, preserved

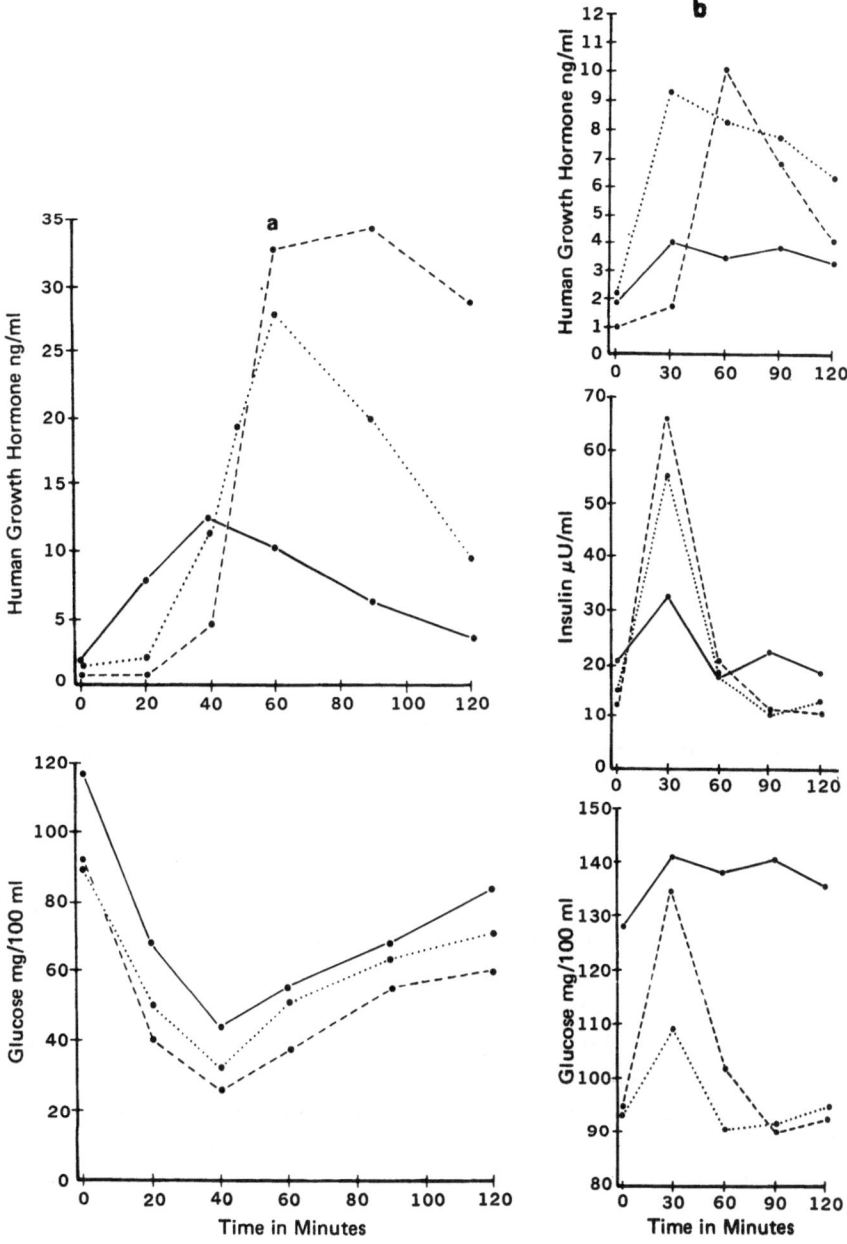

FIGURE 3.11: The response of growth hormone to insulin hypoglycemia (a) or infusion of arginine hydrochloride (b) is blunted during injury, but returns toward normal with recovery. —— Acute burns, ... Recovered burns, ––– Normal man.

Table 3.7   Some Effects of Growth Hormone

Protein metabolism
  1. Growth — increased protein synthesis
     a. nitrogen storage
     b. phosphorus storage
     c. potassium storage
     d. decreased urea excretion
  2. Increased intracellular transport of amino acids
  3. Increased ribosomal protein synthesis
Fat metabolism
  1. Intracellular lipolysis
  2. Increased plasma free fatty acids
  3. Increased oxidation of fat
  4. Ketogenesis stimulated in diabetes
Carbohydrate metabolism
  1. Diminution of insulin responsiveness (aggravation of human diabetes)
  2. Decreased conversion of glucose to fat in adipose tissue
Mineral metabolism
  1. Hypercalciuria
  2. Sodium retention
  3. Phosphorus retention
  4. Hyperphosphatemia
  5. Increased alkaline phosphatase
Effects on connective tissue
  1. Stimulation of chondroitin sulfate synthesis
  2. Stimulation of collagen synthesis
  3. Increased urinary hyroxyproline

Adapted from: Daughaday, W. H., and Parker, M. L.: Human pituitary growth hormone. *Ann. Rev., Med.,* 16:47, 1965.

protoplasmic mass and improved nitrogen retention in the catabolic phase of injury in critically ill burned patients.[33] The protein-sparing effects and enhanced recovery of the injured patients appeared to be dose-related, to require adequate nutrient loading, and to be mediated by alterations of carbohydrate metabolism in the presence of augmented insulin production. In contrast, growth hormone has been administered to starved or injured persons receiving an inadequate caloric intake and nitrogen sparing does not occur. Adequate calories appear necessary for expression of the anticatabolic effect of growth hormone.

[33]Wilmore, D. W., Moylan, J. A., Jr., Bristow, B. F., Mason, A. D., Jr., and Pruitt, B. A., Jr.: Anabolic effects of human growth hormone and high caloric feedings following thermal injury. *Surg. Gynecol. Obstet., 138:875, 1974.*

3.32   IS THYROID HORMONE AN ANABOLIC OR A CATABOLIC AGENT? WHAT IS ITS FUNCTION?

Myxedematous patients usually gain weight while individuals with thyrotoxicosis are hypermetabolic and may lose weight. However, the classification of thyroid hormone as an anabolic or catabolic hormone depends on the dose at which it is administered, as well as the metabolic state of the organism at the time of hormonal administration. The anabolic effects of the hormone are clearly seen in a newborn animal in which thyroidectomy results in a reduction of muscle mass, carcass protein, and protein content of the liver and kidneys. Small amounts of thyroid hormone allow normal growth and development to proceed. In contrast, administration of a large dose of thyroid to the adult animal results in catabolism, characterized by increased excretion of urinary nitrogen, hypermetabolism, and weight loss.

Thyroid hormone stimulates protein synthesis; increased liver mitochondrial protein synthesis appears to be one of the early effects of administered thyroid hormone. Thyroid hormone causes an increased incorporation of labeled RNA precursor into the muscle cell, increased production of messenger RNA, and increased formation of polysomes. Excess administration of T_4 causes loss of protein from muscle, but increased incorporation into liver protein. Continual administration reduces both the liver and carcass protein stores. Cholesterol levels fall with thyroid administration, and this decrease is correlated closely with the rise in basal metabolic rate. The mechanism for the increase in oxygen consumption is not known, but thyroxin requires about 10 days before its peak effect on BMR is seen while triiodothyronine exerts its peak effect 24—36 hr after administration.

3.33   IS T_3 OR T_4 A STRESS HORMONE?

Although it has been proposed that the hypothalamic—pituitary axis acts to stimulate the thyroid following acute stress, there is little evidence to support this claim. Initially, adrenal corticosteroids suppress thyroid elaboration of T_4 although there appears to be a breakthrough of this inhibition after 5—7 days. After T_4 is liberated from the thyroid gland, it is converted in the periphery to a more active iodinated compound, T_3. The liver probably plays a major role in this deiodination step. However, other similar compounds may be formed from T_4, and one which has recently been investigated is reversed T_3 (3,3',5'triiodothyronine), which increases with fasting, operation,[34] or severe trauma,[35] and is elevated in patients with liver disease and in newborn infants. rT_3 is a relatively inactive form of thyroid hormone and decreases further elaboration of thyroid hormone through feedback mechanisms. As T_3 decreases, the effect of the thyroid in heat production and protein synthesis appears to decrease following starvation and liver disease as if compensating to diminish metabolic activity. The sudden decrease in T_3 following starvation is associated with increased gluconeogenesis and may be reversed by carbohydrate intake.[36] A similar decrease in T_3 is observed following elective operation and severe injury.

[34]Burr, W. A., Griffiths, R. S., Black, E. G., and Hoffenberg, R.: Serum triiodothyronine and reverse triiodothyronine concentrations after surgical operations. *Lancet,* 2:1277, 1975.

[35]Becker, R., Johnson, D. W., Woeber, K. A., and Wilmore, D. W.: Decreased serum triiodothyronine (T_3) following thermal injury. *Fed. Proc., 35*:216, 1976.

[36]Spaulding, S. W., Chopra, I. J., Sherwin, R. S., and Lyall, S. S.: Effect of caloric restriction and dietary composition in serum T_3 and reversed T_3 in man. *J. Clin. Endocr. Metab., 42*:197, 1976.

CHAPTER 4

Alterations in Intermediary Metabolism

4.1 WHAT EVENTS FOLLOW INGESTION OF A MEAL?

Man is a meal-eater. During periods of food intake, energy consumption usually exceeds energy expenditure and the additional fuel is stored to be mobilized and utilized during the postabsorptive period. With the consumption of a mixed diet containing fat, carbohydrate, and protein, carbohydrate serves as the primary fuel and triglycerides are primarily stored as adipose tissue. The substance which mediates this response is insulin, although glucagon suppression may also contribute to substrate storage. Excess dietary carbohydrate may also be converted to depot fat if glycogen stores are full. Dietary protein contributes to the maintenance of body structure; the excess amino acids are oxidized in the liver and converted to urea. Protein is not primarily stored as a body fuel, but dietary nitrogen is utilized to rebuild deficits of body protein if they exist.

The body has the unique ability to adapt to large variations in the composition of the food ingested. For example, a high-fat diet induces tissues to increase their capacity to catabolize fat and reduce glucose oxidation. High-carbohydrate diets induce biochemical pathways favoring carbohydrate utilization and fat biosynthesis.

4.2   HOW DOES THE BODY STORE ENERGY?

Energy can be stored in the body in three forms: carbohydrate, protein, and fat. Carbohydrate is stored as glycogen in the liver and skeletal muscle, but these stores are small, accounting for only 1000–1500 calories. Although glycogen reserves are trivial when compared to other energy deposits, the body avidly maintains these stores except under circumstances of stress — exercise, hypoxia, hypovolemia, injury — when glycogen is utilized as an emergency fuel. Conversion of liver glycogen to glucose is an immediate response to adrenergic discharge during stress, and the rapid and immediate rise of blood glucose is the result of liver glycogenolysis following injury. Physical exercise is the major stimulus for utilization of muscle glycogen, although these stores disappear slowly during starvation. Muscle tissue primarily utilizes muscle glycogen at the site of storage or converts the glucose to lactate. Muscle cannot provide blood glucose from its own glycogen since it lacks the enzyme glucose-6-phosphatase.

Protein is not a primary body fuel reservoir: each molecule of protein serves a specific function as an enzyme or for structural or functional purposes. Moreover, protein is maintained in an aqueous environment and provides only approximately 1 kcal/g biological tissue (in contrast to 4 kcal/g yielded by nonhydrated protein). This accounts for the relative inefficiency of protein as a fuel on a unit weight basis.

Lipid is the ideal body fuel. It is stored in an intracellular nonaqueous environment and yields almost 9 kcal/g, which is the caloric value of pure triglyceride. Fat is the critical light-weight, high-energy fuel which is essential to mobile species, carrying their endogenous energy supply.

Man thus has two major energy depots to draw from, protein and fat (Table 4.1). Protein is vital to the structure and function of

Table 4.1   Estimated Fuel Composition of Normal Man

	kg	kcal
Tissues		
Fat	15	141,000
Protein	6	24,000
Glycogen (muscle)	0.150	600
Glycogen (liver)	0.075	300
Total		165,900
Circulating		
Glucose (extracellular water)	0.020	80
Free fatty acids (plasma)	0.0003	3
Triglycerides (plasma)	0.003	30
Total		113

Adapted from: Cahill, G. F., Jr.: Starvation in man. *New Eng. J. Med.,* *282*:668, 1970.

the body and mechanisms are available for conservation. Although fat has other minor functions, it primarily represents the major energy reservoir for man.

4.3   HOW DOES MAN RESPOND TO SHORT-TERM STARVATION? WHAT IS THE CORI CYCLE?

The body readily responds to the absence of food by neural— hormonal alterations which mobilize substrate from peripheral fuel deposits. After 18—24 hr of fasting, liver glycogen and muscle amino acids, converted in the liver to new glucose, provide an ongoing supply of glucose for glycolytic tissue. The brain and nervous tissue utilize approximately 80% of the daily hepatic production of glucose and completely oxidize the fuel to CO_2 and water. Other tissues that require glucose (red cell, white cell, bone marrow, renal medulla) or partially utilize glucose (skeletal muscle) convert the glucose to lactate and pyruvate and release these intermediates into the blood stream where they are reconverted in the liver to new glucose. This process of glucose conservation is the "Cori cycle." This cycle describes an energy shuttle system which starts with a molecule of hepatic glucose which is transferred to peripheral tissue, converted to two molecules of lactate (energy-yielding), and is then recycled to the liver to be reconverted to new glucose (energy-requiring). The energy required for hepatic gluconeogenesis is derived primarily from the oxidation of fat in the liver; thus, fat shares (or shuttles) its stored energy with glycolytic tissues which cannot primarily oxidize fat. In addition, gluconeogenesis from protein is spared by limiting complete oxidation of glucose to CO_2 and water. While gluconeogenesis provides fuel for specialized tissues, the remainder of the body oxidizes fatty acids released directly into the circulation or partially oxidized in the liver to "ketone bodies" (acetoacetate or β-hydroxybutyrate). Tissues which can utilize glucose (such as skeletal muscle) shift to fat oxidation, and the glucose that enters these tissues is converted to lactate and sent back to the liver. Thus, the need for glucose is minimized and protein is further spared.

4.4   WHAT CAUSES "KETOSIS"? IS IT BENEFICIAL? . . . HARMFUL?

If carbohydrate is omitted from the diet, insulin secretion impaired, or total starvation undertaken, fatty acid mobilization and utilization are favored at very high rates of oxidation. Increased concentrations of fatty acid impede glucose entry into muscle cells and therefore act as potent peripheral glucose antagonists.[1] Within several days of starvation, fatty acids will be partially oxidized in the liver to form acetylacetate, acetone, or β-hydroxybutyrate compounds which are known as "ketone bodies." The parent body of ketones, acetoacetyl CoA, is a normal intermediate of lipogenesis and fatty acid degradation, and fatty acid oxidation appears unimpaired to the level at which acetyl CoA is formed. For acetyl CoA to be utilized in the citric acid cycle, it must combine with oxaloacetate, which is an end-product of carbohydrate breakdown, arising from the conversion of pyruvate to oxaloacetate. However, with glucose availability impaired or limited (either by starvation or by diabetes), the citric acid cycle is rate-limited by the diminished amount of oxaloacetate present and hence fatty acid breakdown is shunted by way of CoA into ketone-body formation (Fig. 4.1). During starvation, ketones are the main source of body fuel, and either directly or indirectly

[1] Randle, P. J., Hales, C. N., Garland, P. B., and Newsholme, E. A.: The glucose fatty-acid cycle. Its role in insulin sensitivity and the metabolic disturbance of diabetes mellitus. *Lancet, 1*:785, 1963.

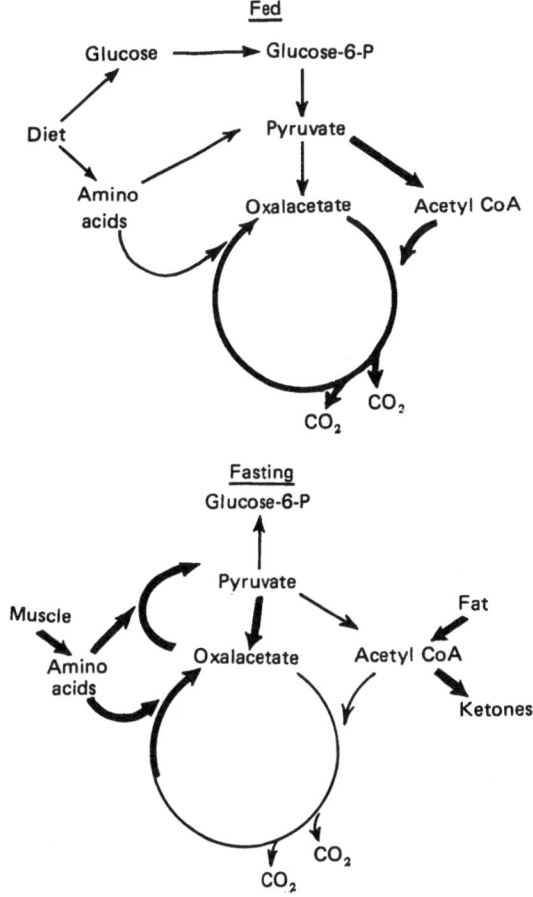

FIGURE 4.1: The flow of substrate during the fed and fasting states.

provide the signal to muscle cells to minimize amino acid release, which aids protein conservation during long-term caloric deprivation. During ketosis, the fat breakdown products appear in the blood and urine, and urine ketones represent an overflow of fatty acid catabolites that are not extracted by fat-utilizing tissue, primarily skeletal muscle.

Ketonemia and ketonuria are accompanied by mild metabolic acidosis. This is usually compensated for and of little consequence unless the subject is stressed, and then buffer capacity is limited. Progressive acidosis may account in part for the decreased aerobic work capacity, diminished physical fitness scores, and altered cardio-vascular response to exercise observed in patients on high-fat diets or in starvation ketosis.[2] Ketosis in the uncontrolled diabetic is ac-companied by concomitant salt and water losses, hypovolemia, and hyperosmolality as a result of an osmotic diuresis resulting from the hyperglycemia.

4.5   HOW DO THE BLOOD SUBSTRATES CHANGE DURING FASTING? HOW DOES THIS REFLECT ALTERATIONS IN OXIDIZED FUELS?

As fasting progresses, alterations in the concentrations of key circu-lating substrates occur: blood glucose falls, free fatty acids and ketone bodies rise, and levels of total serum amino acids gradually fall (Table 4.2). These alterations in plasma concentrations generally reflect the decrease in glucose as a primary fuel, and the relative increase in fat oxidation as the body's major energy source (Table 4.3). Studies of serum concentration alone, however, do not clearly demonstrate the entire sequence of metabolic events which occur during adaptation to starvation, and the use of tracer materials and regional catheterization techniques have been necessary to charac-terize the dynamics of substrate flow.

4.6   WHAT HORMONE CONTROLS SUBSTRATE FLOW DURING BRIEF FASTING?

Insulin appears to play a central role in man's adaptation to fasting. As insulin falls, the rate of free fatty acid release is increased. In addition, amino acid release from skeletal muscle is increased, and some of these substances are converted in the liver to new glucose. In the first several days of fasting, catecholamine excretion rate may increase, probably in response to the initial fall in blood glucose.[3]

[2]Lategola, M. T.: The effect of 5-day, complete starvation on cardiopulmonary functions of aerobic work capacity and orthostatic tolerance. *Fed. Proc., 24*:590, 1965.

[3]Misbin, R. I., Edgar, P. J., and Lockwood, D. H.: Influence of adrenergic receptor stimulation on glucose metabolism during starvation in man: effects on circulating levels of insulin, growth hormone and fatty acids. *Metabolism, 20*:544, 1971.

Table 4.2   Alterations in Blood Substrate and Hormones during Fasting
(Mean of Venous Samples from 11 Obese Subjects)

Days of fast:	0	3	10	24	35–38
Glucose (mg/100 ml)	86	65	68	68	67
Free fatty acids (mmol/liter)	0.71	1.25	1.36	1.55	1.60
β-Hydroxybutyrate (mmol/liter)	0.07	1.21	4.30	5.78	5.85
Acetoacetate (mmol/liter)	0.03	0.41	1.00	1.27	1.34
Glycerol (mmol/liter)	0.092	0.108	0.110	0.154	0.124
α-Amino nitrogen (mmol/liter)	4.39	4.32	4.41	3.85	3.85
Insulin (μU/ml)	37	20	20	13	14
Growth hormone (ng/ml)	1.0	1.4	1.2	0.5	0.4

Adapted from: Owen, O. E., Felig, P., Morgan, A. P., Wahren, J., and Cahill, G. F., Jr.: Liver and kidney metabolism during prolonged starvation. *J. Clin. Invest.*, *48*:574, 1969.

Table 4.3   Body Fuels Oxidized during Brief Fasting

Day of fast	Nitrogen excretion (g)	Metabolic rate (kcal)	Fuel metabolized			Percentage of total metabolism		
			Carbohydrate (g)	Protein (g)	Fat (g)	Carbohydrate	Protein	Fat
1	7.1	1663	69	43	135	16.6	10.3	73.1
2	8.4	1646	42	50	142	10.2	12.2	77.6
3	11.3	1598	39	68	130	9.8	17.0	73.2
4	11.9	1524	4	71	136	1.0	18.7	80.3
5	10.4	1449	0	63	133	0	17.4	82.6
6	10.2	1441	0	61	133	0	16.9	83.1
7	9.8	1442	0	59	134	0	16.4	83.6

Adapted from: Peters, J. P., and Van Slyke, D. D.: *Quantitative Clinical Chemistry*, 2nd Ed. Baltimore, Williams & Wilkins Co., 1946, p. 649.

The increased irritability and palpitations which frequently occur on the second to third day of fasting may be clinical manifestations of increased adrenergic discharge. The initial catecholamine discharge may accelerate release of free fatty acid and amino acids, although lack of central autonomic regulation does not appear to alter the initial adaptive response to starvation. Catecholamine levels then fall and remain low throughout the remainder of the fast.[4] Glucagon rises with fasting and the I/G ratio is low, favoring hepatic gluco-

[4]Bourgeois, B., Schmidt, B. J., and Bourgeois, R.: Some aspects of catecholamines in undernutrition. *In* Gardner, L. I., and Amacher, P., (Eds.): *Endocrine Aspects of Malnutrition.* Santa Ynez, the KROC Foundation, 1973, p. 163.

neogenesis. Other hormones, such as ACTH, TSH, and growth hormone, are altered but are of minor importance in the overall adaptation.

4.7   HOW DOES MAN ADAPT TO LONGER PERIODS OF STARVATION? WHAT IS THE TIME COURSE FOR STARVATION ADAPTATION?

1. *Reduces Energy Expenditure.* There is a gradual decrease in total body energy expenditure. The fall in metabolic rate is proportionately greater than loss of total body mass (see p. 33).

2. *Conserves Protein.* There is a gradual decrease in urinary nitrogen (primarily urea) which plateaus as low as 3—5 g/day between the second and third week (Fig. 4.2). The proportion of energy obtained from nitrogen at this time is constant and represents between 15 and 18% of the metabolic fuel oxidized (Table 4.4). As previously noted, the mechanisms for adaptation appear to be utilization of ketone bodies by skeletal muscle and gradual adaptation of the brain to oxidize fat as a partial fuel, thus decreasing some of the requirement for proteolysis and gluconeogenesis. Studies in animals and man suggest that the initial adaptation to low or no protein intake occurs by an alteration or diversion of amino acid pathways away from urea formation,

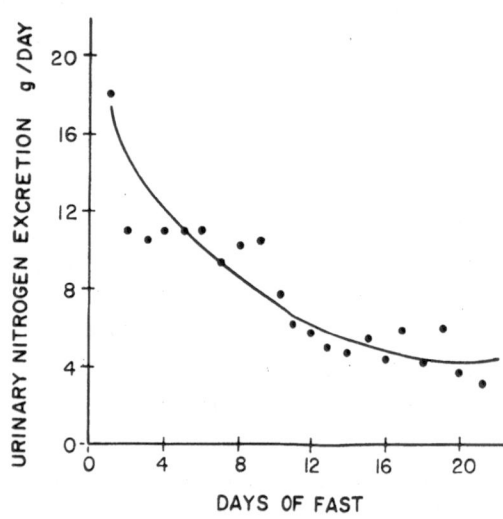

FIGURE 4.2: The decreased nitrogen excretion which occurs with a prolonged fast. Adapted from Freund, E. and Freund, O.: Beiträge zum Stoffwechsel in Hunger-Zustande. *Wiener Klinische Rundshau, 15*:91, 1901.

Table 4.4

Days of fast	Weight at start of each period (kg)	Urinary nitrogen (g/day)	Calorie expenditure (kcal/day)	Calories from nitrogen (%)
3 preliminary days	–	14.0	–	–
1–7	60.6	9.9	1650	15
8–14	55.1	10.3	1450	18
15–21	52.8	8.4	1290	17
22–28	50.1	7.8	1250	16
29–31	48.1	7.2	1260	15

Adapted from: Peters, J. P., and Van Slyke, D. D.: *Quantitative Clinical Chemistry*, 2nd Ed. Baltimore, Williams & Wilkins Co., 1946, p. 648.

reducing urea excretion but maintaining normal body protein turnover. With time, total body protein turnover is reduced. Synthesis of albumin is closely related to protein intake, and intravascular albumin mass is also preserved by mechanisms which transfer albumin from the extravascular to the intravascular pool. The mechanisms for adaptation to alterations in protein content of the diet reside in the liver. Amino acid activating enzymes increase while there is a decrease in the urea cycle enzymes, favoring incorporation of amino acids into protein[5] and shunting amino acids away from urea formation. Finally, there may be alterations in enzymatic adaptations in various organs. For example, it appears that liver protein synthesis is initially maintained in rats placed on low-protein or protein-free diets, while the rate of synthesis is rapidly reduced in skeletal muscle. With time, there is a generalized reduction in protein synthesis throughout the body.

3. *Utilization of Ketone Bodies by the Brain.* With time, the central nervous system shifts to fat as its major fuel source although it still continues to utilize a major portion of the body's glucose. Ketone bodies are water-insoluble, and can readily enter the central nervous system for oxidation. As the brain shifts to ketone utilization, gluconeogenesis and urea excretion fall to their nadir.

[5]Waterlow, J. C.: Observations on the mechanism of adaptation to low protein intakes. *Lancet*, 2:1091, 1968.

4.8   ARE RENAL FUNCTION AND METABOLISM AFFECTED DURING PROLONGED STARVATION?

During prolonged starvation, the kidney becomes a significant source of new glucose, contributing almost half of the body glucose after 30 days of fasting. During early starvation, about 90% of the gluco-neogenesis occurs in the liver and only 10% arises from the kidney. After prolonged starvation, urea is no longer the major nitrogen excretory product, and its place is taken by ammonia (Fig. 4.3). This adaptive mechanism occurs in the kidney as ammonia accepts hydrogen ion for excretion in order to compensate for acidic metabolic end products. Approximately 100 mEq/day of base would be required to neutralize the excreted keto acid each day, which would require exogenous intake of a fixed base or metabolic production of base if this compensatory mechanism were not available.

A unique mechanism utilizing muscle glutamine as the shuttle carrier supports renal ammonia production, which compensates for

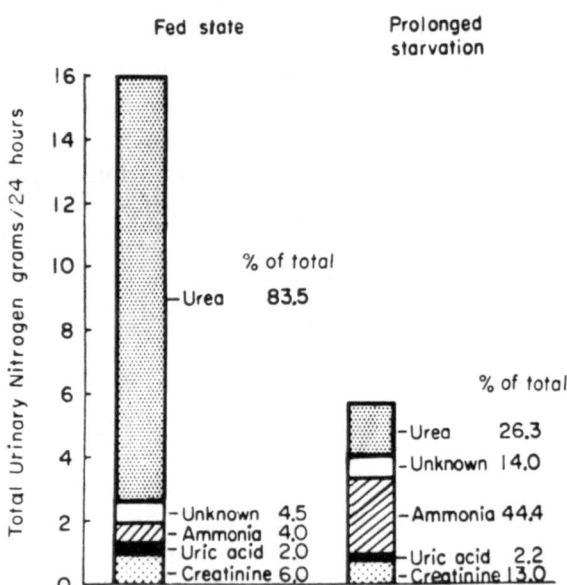

FIGURE 4.3: Urinary nitrogen excretion components. Adapted from: Owen, O. E., Felig, P., Morgan, A. P., Wahren, J., and Cahill, G. F., Jr.: Liver and kidney metabolism during prolonged starvation. *J. Clin. Invest.*, *48*:574, 1969.

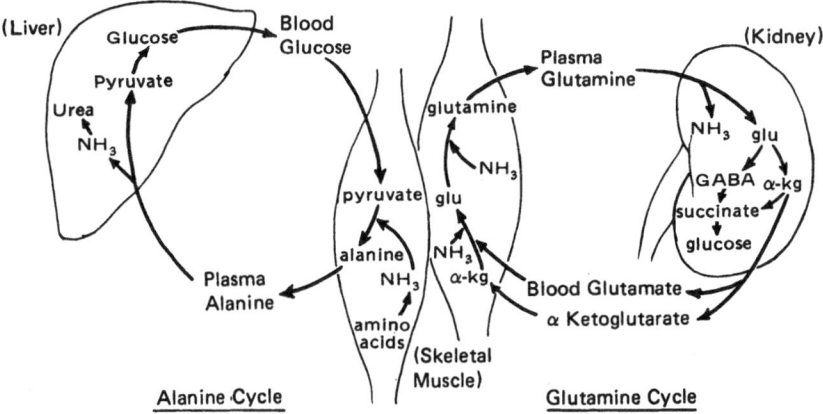

FIGURE 4.4: Two cycles are thought to shuttle carbon chains and ammonia from skeletal muscle to visceral tissues. Liver and kidney extract both alanine and glutamine; in this diagram, kidney is shown participating in the "glutamine cycle" while liver participates in the "alanine cycle." Adapted from: Scriver, C. R., and Rosenberg, L. E.: *Amino Acid Metabolism and Its Disorders*. Philadelphia, W. B. Saunders, 1973, p. 83.

the metabolic acid end-products. The kidney is the recipient of muscle glutamine (Fig. 4.4). The glutamine is deaminated to provide ammonia and the end-product, glutamate, may accept additional ammonia, be utilized for purposes of synthesis, or, following deamination, contribute to the pool of new glucose. Thus, the kidney neutralizes the acid load and simultaneously produces new glucose for the body.

4.9   WHAT IS THE ALANINE CYCLE?

Some of the amino acids released from skeletal muscle serve as three-carbon precursors for glucose, similar to lactate and pyruvate from the Cori cycle, and glycerol which arises from triglyceride breakdown. The major gluconeogenic amino acid, alanine, is released from muscle in greater quantities than are stored in skeletal muscle protein. Biochemical studies suggest that the three-carbon skeleton for alanine arises in the muscle from pyruvate, which accepts nitrogen by transamination from the branched-chain amino acids, leucine, isoleucine, and valine. The branched-chain amino acids are not processed in the liver but pass through the splanchnic circulation and are oxidized in skeletal muscle. Addition of branched-chain amino acids to *in vitro* muscle preparations results in increased protein synthesis and inhibited degradation.[6]

The alanine shuttle system is thought to represent another form of ammonia transport from the periphery to liver. Peripheral oxidation of branched-chain amino acids would cause a rise of ammonia in the blood if a bound carrier system were not available. This shuttle system carries the ammonia in bound form and provides a three-carbon skeleton that is utilized as a substrate for glucose. The nitrogen residue is converted to urea for excretion. Other amino acids that serve as significant gluconeogenic precursors are listed in Table 4.5.

Table 4.5   Arterial-Hepatic Venous Differences of Some Gluconeogenic Amino Acids after Starvation (Mean μ Mol/Liter)

	Postabsorptive ($n = 5$)	Brief fast (36–48 hr; $n = 3$)	Prolonged fast (5–6 weeks; $n = 4$)
Threonine	24.3	42.3	14.7
Serine	31.5	43.3	25.9
Glycine	40.9	68.0	7.6
Alanine	120.6	232.3	59.5
Valine	13.5	43.5	9.7
Methionine	4.5	10.2	5.2
Tyrosine	12.3	15.2	10.4
Phenylalanine	9.4	12.1	8.4

Adapted from: Felig, P., Owen, O. E., Wahren, J., and Cahill, G. F., Jr.: Amino acid metabolism during prolonged starvation. *J. Clin. Invest.*, *48*:584, 1969.

4.10   HOW IS THE NITROGEN LOST DURING STARVATION AFFECTED BY GLUCOSE? BY INGESTION OF AMINO ACIDS? ... OF FATS?

In his classic "life raft" studies, Gamble noted that the intake of 100 g of glucose per day resulted in a prompt decrease in urinary nitrogen excretion during the starved state.[7] This small amount of

[6]Fulks, R. M., Li, J. B., and Goldberg, A. L.: Effects of insulin, glucose, and amino acids on protein turnover in rat diaphragm. *J. Biol. Chem.*, *250*:290, 1975.
[7]Gamble, J. L.: *Chemical Anatomy, Physiology and Pathology of Extracellular Fluid: A Lecture Syllabus*, 5th Ed. Cambridge, Mass., Harvard University Press, 1947.

glucose stimulates insulin elaboration which limits proteolysis and gluconeogenesis. Insulin also decreases ketogenesis. The ingested glucose is utilized by glycolytic tissues while the remainder of the body continues to oxidize fats. Infusion of 400–700 g of carbohydrate per day markedly diminishes nitrogen loss by signaling for increased insulin elaboration.[8]

After an appropriate period of adaptation, amino acids appear to blunt the nitrogen loss that occurs with starvation. In obese individuals undergoing weight reduction, nitrogen balance was enhanced by feeding 55 g of amino acid each day after 2–3 weeks of starvation.[9]

Fat ingestion during starvation maintains the body triglyceride stores but does not alter nitrogen conservation that cannot be explained by starvation adaptation alone.[10]

4.11   WHAT ARE THE BODY COMPOSITIONAL CHANGES THAT OCCUR DURING PARTIAL OR TOTAL STARVATION?

With starvation or semistarvation, there is a gradual increase in the extracellular fluid, a disproportionate loss of fat, loss of metabolically active tissue (lean body mass), and maintenance of bone and connective tissue.

These compositional alterations reflect the protein conservation that occurs and the utilization of fat as a caloric source, which accounts for approximately 85% of the energy oxidized by the body. The caloric value of the tissue lost in early starvation is much lower than observed in prolonged starvation. The caloric equivalent of the lost tissue is approximately 2000 kcal/kg in early starvation and gradually increases to 8000 kcal/kg as starvation progresses.[11] This

[8] O'Connell, R. C., Morgan, A. P., Aoki, T. T., Ball, M. R., and Moore, F. D.: Nitrogen conservation in starvation: graded response to intravenous glucose. *J. Clin. Endocr. Metab.*, 39:555, 1974.

[9] Apfelbaum, M., Bostsarron, J., and Brigant, L.: La diminution de la consommation "basale" d'oxygène sous l'effet d'une restriction calorique chez du sujets en bilan d'azote equilibre. *Rev. Franc. Etud., Clin. Biol.*, 14:361, 1969.

[10] Brennan, M. F., Fitzpatrick, G. F., Cohen, K. H., and Moore, F. D.: Glycerol: major contributor to the short term protein sparing effect of fat emulsions in normal man. *Ann. Surg.*, 182:386, 1975.

[11] Grande, F.: Energetics and weight reduction. *Amer. J. Clin. Nutr.*, 21:305, 1968.

alteration in the caloric content of oxidized fuel demonstrates the gradual adjustment which occurs as the body shifts predominantly to fat utilization (fat yielding approximately 8000 kcal/kg body fat).

4.12   WHAT ARE SOME OF THE ALTERATIONS IN ORGAN COMPOSITION FOLLOWING STARVATION?

Porter reported on organ weight obtained from 459 autopsies of individuals that had died of starvation.[12] The greatest weight losses were found in the pancreas, spleen, kidney, liver, genitals, gut, blood, and muscles, and the least in the skeleton and eyes. Others have assessed the protein content in the organs of animals following a brief or prolonged fast and have shown that the liver and pancreas lose the most protein, but significant protein loss occurred from the prostate, seminal vesicles, gastrointestinal tract, and kidney. The skeleton and brain appear reasonably well protected.[13]

4.13   WHAT IMPORTANT PHYSIOLOGICAL CONSEQUENCES ARE ASSOCIATED WITH SEMI- OR TOTAL STARVATION?

There are a wide variety of physiological limitations that result from food deprivation and their major consequences[14] are summarized below:

1. *Gastrointestinal Function.* Diarrhea, nonspecific dysentery, colic, flatulence, and a protruding abdomen are universally recognized symptoms during states of energy deprivation. Gastric emptying and intestinal motility are depressed, and these alterations have been related to visceral edema, and reversed by albumin administration.[15] Gastric acidity may be reduced, exocrine pancreatic secretion insufficient, and small-bowel absorption impaired, an

---

[12]Porter, A.: *The Disease of the Madras Famine of 1877–78.* Madras, India, Government Press, 1889.

[13]Addis, T., Poo, L. J., and Lew, W.: The quantities of protein lost by the various organs and tissues of the body during a fast. *J. Biol. Chem.*, 115:111, 1936.

[14]Keys, A., Brožek, J., Henschel, A., Mickelsen, O., and Taylor, H. L.: *The Biology of Human Starvation*, Vol. 1. Minneapolis, University of Minnesota Press, 1950.

[15]Mecray, P. M., Barden, R. P., and Ravdin, I. S.: Nutritional edema: its effect on gastric emptying time before and after gastric operations. *Surgery*, 1:53, 1937.

absorptive deficit associated with intestinal villous atrophy. In spite of these alterations, the vast majority of famine victims take nourishment by mouth without special difficulty.

2. *Circulation and Cardiac Function.* Bradycardia, hypotension, occasional vertigo, slight cyanosis, and electrocardiographic abnormalities are frequently observed in starved individuals. Cardiac output is decreased, and this reduction appears somewhat greater than the reduction in metabolic rate. Normal cardiocirculatory function returns slowly with nutrition repletion, and the starved patient has reduced cardiac reserve; heart failure has been observed with sudden overeating or with administration of intravenous salt or other volume loads.

3. *Respiration.* Vital capacity is decreased probably due to a reduction in the strength of the respiratory musculature. Respiratory efficiency (milliliters of oxygen utilized per liter of inspired oxygen) also falls and this effect is most marked when metabolic demands are increased, during exercise or critical illness.

4. *Work Capacity.* The capacity of the individual to accomplish physical work decreases with progressive undernutrition: weakness is a cardinal symptom of starvation. Physical capacity may be limited not only by lack of fuel, but also by the performance of the circulatory, respiratory, and neuromuscular systems. Work capacity improves with refeeding and physical rehabilitation.

4.14   WHAT IS THE RELATIONSHIP BETWEEN INFECTIOUS DISEASE AND UNDERNUTRITION?

"From time immemorial, famine and pestilence have been considered an inseparable pair, the twin fruits of war, but inseparable also when famine occurs without man's being the sole creator of his misfortune."[16] Now, this inseparable pair, malnutrition and infection, serve as the major cause of death in hospitalized, critically ill patients. Factors which may contribute to this interaction are summarized below:

1. *Impairment of the Barrier Function of Membranes.* Malnutrition alters metabolic rate in various tissues, and cellular turnover in

[16]Keys, A., Brožek, J., Henschel, A., Mickelsen, O., and Taylor, H. L.: *The Biology of Human Starvation*, Vol. 2. Minneapolis, University of Minnesota Press, 1950, p. 1002.

skin and the gastrointestinal mucosa may be depressed. The barrier function of these surfaces may diminish as the membranes become more permeable; ingested bacteria appear more rapidly in the blood stream and lymph nodes in animals following fasting. Endogenous flora which normally reside in the intestinal tract account for the majority of infections in critically ill patients, and the route of entry to the body across the gut has been associated with specific procedures which compromise the barrier function of the gut. Intraluminal treatment of *Candida albicans* has been proposed as an adjunctive treatment for systemic candidiasis.

2. *Alteration in Body Temperature.* Body and surface temperature are $1-2°C$ cooler in malnourished individuals than in normals and the febrile response to infection is frequently diminished. The ability to generate increased body temperature has been related to host defense capability to resist infection, and this response may be impaired in the malnourished patient.

3. *Antibody Production.* Paul Cannon emphasized the relationship between protein intake and antibody production, and demonstrated a decrease in the production of agglutinins after immunization of specific antigenic agents in protein deficient animals.[17] A similar attenuation in the antibody response was observed by Gell in man following injection of tobacco mosaic virus and avian red cells.[18] Discrepancies in both of these reports have been noted, and it is uncertain at what point protein deficiency is critical for antibody production; this relationship may be clearly observed with prolonged malnutrition and extreme deficiency.

4. *Cellular Immunity.* Impairment of the responses to a variety of skin tests have been reported in malnourished patients. Peripheral blood lymphocytes obtained from malnourished persons and cultured *in vitro* demonstrate depressed proliferative response to phytohemagglutinin. In hypoalbuminic patients with normal levels of serum immunoglobulins A, G, and M, peripheral blood

[17]Cannon, P. R., Chase, W. E., and Wissler, R. W.: The relationship of the protein reserves to antibody production. I. The effects of a low protein diet and of plasmapheresis upon the formation of agglutinins. *J. Immunol.*, 47:133, 1943.

[18]Gell, P. G. H.: Discussion of nutrition and resistance to infection. *Proc. R. Soc. Med.*, 41:323, 1948.

lymphocytes responded poorly to *in vitro* stimulation. Skin test reactivity and lymphocyte proliferative response improved significantly following 2–3 weeks of nutritional repletion.[19]

4.15   HOW DO THE METABOLIC EVENTS CHANGE WITH TIME FOLLOWING INJURY OR INFECTION?

Immediately after the injury, there may be depression of physiological responses to hormonal discharge, which may be transitory and a manifestation of circulatory inadequacy or neurogenic shock. Cuthbertson[20] refers to this early phase as the "ebb" phase of injury. If blood volume is restored, adequate oxygen provided, and sufficient circulation reestablished, the organism usually survives. The early "ebb" phase response is then generally followed by an increase in metabolic reactions ("flow" phase), presumably to provide substrate for inflammatory reactions and tissue repair.

Moore[21] categorized surgical convalescence into four phases, which seem to reflect gradual recovery during the "flow" phase of injury.

1. The first phase: characterized by the catabolic response to injury.
2. The turning point: once referred to as the "corticoid-withdrawal" phase, observed 3–7 days following moderate-sized operations, and characterized by the patient spontaneously saying "I feel better today."
3. Gain in muscle strength: as the patient becomes anabolic, his caloric intake and activity increase and he regains muscle strength and retains nitrogen. This may continue for 2–5 weeks, depending on the extent of the catabolic response to the initial injury.

[19]Law, D. K., Dudrick, S. J., and Abdon, N. I.: Immunocompetence of patients with protein–calorie malnutrition. The effect of nutritional repletion. *Ann. Int. Med.,* 79:545, 1973.

[20]Cuthbertson, D., and Tilstone, W. J.: Metabolism during the postinjury period. *Adv. Clin. Chem.,* 12:1, 1969.

[21]Moore, F. D.: *Metabolic Care of the Surgical Patient.* Philadelphia, W. B. Saunders, 1959, p. 28.

4. Fat gain: usually observed after the patient has been discharged from the hospital and returns for an office visit. Restoration of body fat is the final signal that the patient is returning to normal body composition.

4.16   WHAT FACTORS DIRECT THE METABOLIC RESPONSE TO INJURY? ... TO INFECTION?

A variety of factors may elicit the metabolic response to injury. Immediate sympathetic discharge results from direct injury to the central nervous system, hypoxia or anoxia due to airway injury or obstruction, decreased blood volume, and pain or anxiety. Once these acute alterations in homeostasis are managed effectively, other factors such as the cross-sectional mass of tissue injured, loss of normal barriers to infection, and starvation contribute to the catabolic stress response to injury. As previously noted (p. 83), denervation of the wound or interruption of sensory input to the brain has not altered the hypermetabolic response during the "flow" phase of injury.

Blood-borne mediators have been specifically associated with the metabolic response to infection (p. 70). These substances may be products of the offending organisms (endotoxins) or liberated as a response of the host cells to the infection. Endogenous pyrogen and leukocyte endogenous mediator (LEM) may be elaborated with phagocytosis (Fig. 4.5). While both substances may produce a fever, LEM has specific actions in the liver to promote hepatic uptake of plasma zinc and iron, increase plasma copper (ceruloplasmin), and stimulate hepatic uptake of plasma amino acids which are utilized in the synthesis of acute-phase globulins.[22] Thus, a specific inflammatory cell may regulate body redistribution of trace elements and nitrogen and stimulate acute-phase globulin synthesis to participate in the host defense mechanisms.

[22]Wannemacher, R. W., Jr., DuPont, H. L., Pekarek, R. S., Powanda, M. C., Schwartz, A., Hornick, R. B., and Beisel, W. R.: An endogenous mediator of depression of amino acids and trace metals in serum during typhoid fever. *J. Infect. Dis., 126*:77, 1972.

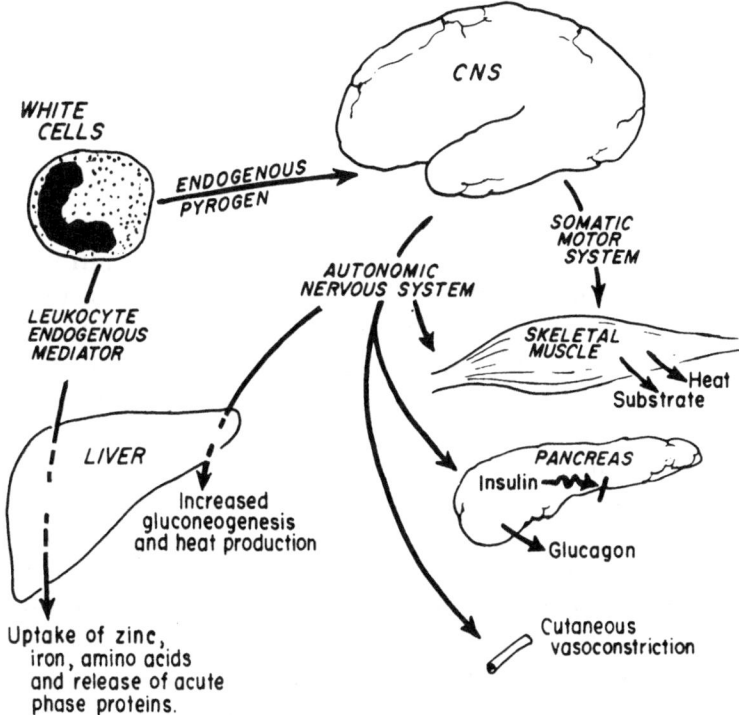

FIGURE 4.5: Pyrogens liberated by cells involved in the inflammatory reaction influence a variety of physiologic responses by altering hypothalamic temperature "setpoint" or acting directly on the liver to affect hepatic metabolism.

4.17 WHAT ARE THE CHARACTERISTIC METABOLIC ALTERATIONS WHICH ARE ASSOCIATED WITH INJURY AND SURGICAL INFECTION?

1. *Diminished Protein Economy.* Urinary nitrogen excretion is increased compared to normal man receiving the same intake of calories and nitrogen.
2. *Hypermetabolism.* Increase in basal oxygen consumption.
3. *Altered Glucose Kinetics.* Changes in hepatic production and peripheral uptake of glucose that account for alterations in fasting serum glucose concentrations and disappearance of glucose following a carbohydrate load.
4. *Loss of Body Weight and Erosion of Lean Body Mass.* The consequences of the responses listed above that may be blunted or reversed by adequate nutrition.

4.18   WHAT ARE THE ROUTES OF PROTEIN LOSS FROM THE BODY FOLLOWING TRAUMA OR INFECTION?

At the turn of this century, increased loss of body protein was described in patients with infectious diseases, and during World War I, acceleration of protein catabolism was described as a metabolic consequence of injury. Yet, it was not until Cuthbertson and associates demonstrated the increased urinary loss of nitrogen and other intracellular constituents following long-bone fracture that alterations in protein economy became a recognized feature of the posttraumatic metabolic response to injury. Following moderate to severe trauma in otherwise healthy adults, there is a marked rise in urinary nitrogen, sulfur, phosphorus, potassium, magnesium, zinc, and creatine, all substances that reside in the cell. The rise in urinary nitrogen is primarily an increase in urea, which comprises approximately 80—90% of the total urinary nitrogen. Abnormal protein loss from the gastrointestinal tract does not occur, and most patients with previously normal intestinal function, receiving hospital diets, lose less than 2 g of nitrogen per day in their stools unless diarrhea is present. However, protein loss from an open wound is significant and burn-wound loss contributes approximately 20—25% of the total nitrogen lost from the body in the early postburn period, with surface losses decreasing in time and returning to normal with closure of the burn wound.[23] Wound loss represents only a fraction of the total nitrogen lost from the body, and the mechanism of protein leakage through the wound is distinctly different from the hypercatabolic process which depletes body protein stores.

4.19   WHERE DOES THE PROTEIN EXCRETED IN THE URINE ORIGINATE?

When Cuthbertson concluded his earlier studies on protein catabolism following injury, he commented that the nitrogen subsequently lost from the body came from systemic stores rather than arising from damaged tissue at the injury site. Others have confirmed this concept, and most evidence suggests that the main source of

[23]Soroff, H. S., Pearson, E., and Artz, C. P.: An estimation of the nitrogen requirements for equilibrium in burned patients. *Surg. Gynecol. Obstet., 112:*159, 1961.

catabolized protein is from skeletal muscle: a conclusion based on the magnitude of nitrogen loss, the clinical evidence of muscle wasting and decreased strength, serial body compositional measurements, and muscle biopsies in humans and carcass analysis in small animals. Recent studies demonstrate increased excretion of 3-methylhistidine in injured and infected patients. This nonmetabolized amino acid arises only from muscle, and its excretion rate closely parallels muscle protein breakdown.

4.20   WHAT DETERMINES THE MAGNITUDE OF THE NITROGEN EXCRETED IN THE URINE? HOW IS THIS RELATED TO OXYGEN CONSUMPTION? ... TO OTHER FACTORS?

Nitrogen loss is related to the size of the injury or extent of infection (Table 4.6), decreases with time, and returns to normal with resolution of the stress.

The extent of nitrogen loss correlates closely with oxygen consumption of the patient; both heat production and nitrogen excretion are related to the extent of stress (Fig. 4.6). Duke and

Table 4.6   Estimates of Nitrogen Loss Following Catabolic Illness (First 10 Days, *ad lib* Feedings)

Precipitating factor	Cumulative nitrogen loss (g)
Injury	
Major burn	170
Multiple injury	150
Peritonitis	136
Simple fracture	115
Major operation	50
Minor operation	24
Infection	
Typhoid fever (untreated)	116
Pneumonia (untreated)	59
Tularemia (treated)	52
Q fever (treated)	40
Sandfly fever (untreated)	16

Adapted in part from: Wannemacher, R. W., Jr.: Protein metabolism (applied biochemistry). *In* H. Ghadimi (Ed.): *Total Parenteral Nutrition: Premises and Promises.* New York, John Wiley, 1975, p. 113.

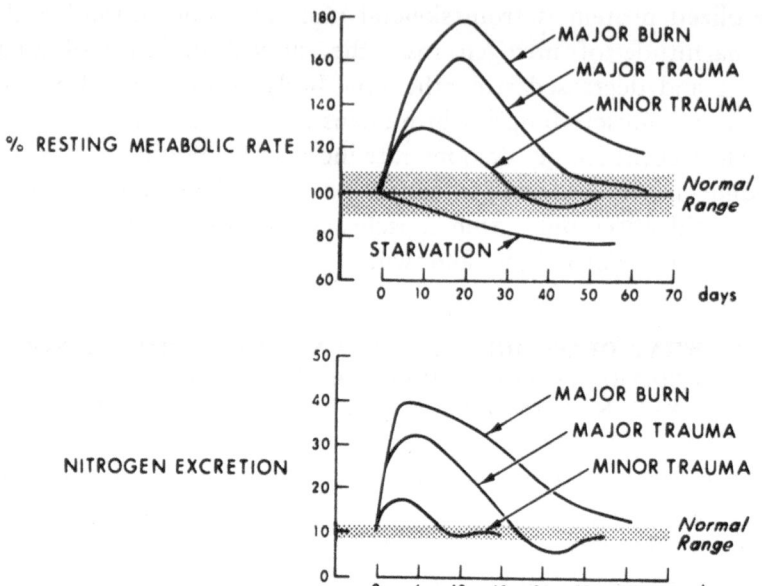

% RESTING METABOLIC RATE

NITROGEN EXCRETION

FIGURE 4.6: Hypermetabolism and increased nitrogen excretion are closely related following minor or major trauma or major burn injury. Patients received 12 g nitrogen intake per day. Adapted from: Kinney, J. M.: Energy deficits in acute illness and injury. *In*: A. P. Morgan (Ed.): *Proceedings of a Conference on Energy Metabolism and Body Fuel Utilization*, Cambridge, Harvard University Press, 1966, p. 174.

associates[24] demonstrated that nitrogen contributes a constant 15–20% of the metabolic fuel oxidized during a variety of catabolic illnesses. The remainder of the metabolic fuel was derived from fat stores. Other factors (bed rest, poor nutritional intake, and a low ambient temperature) are additive to the basic reset in protein catabolism that occurs following injury.

4.21 HOW DO PREINJURY BODY COMPOSITION AND PROTEIN STORES AFFECT THE MAGNITUDE OF THE NITROGEN EXCRETED FOLLOWING STRESS OR STARVATION?

Young muscular and/or athletic individuals excrete much more nitrogen following injury than sedentary or debilitated patients with

[24]Duke, J. H., Jr., Jorgensen, S. B., Broell, J. R., Long, C. L., and Kinney, J. M.: Contribution of protein to caloric expenditure following injury. *Surgery*, *68*:168, 1970.

reduced protein stores. Johnson[25] contrasted the quantity of nitrogen loss in a group of well-nourished individuals undergoing gastric operations with a group of poorly nourished patients requiring proctocolectomy. Despite the fact that the proctocolectomy patients were subject to a more traumatic operation and greater surgical stress, their nitrogen losses were substantially less, emphasizing the relationship between the nutritional state of the patient and the posttraumatic responses. Women, with their slightly increased body fat mass and diminished lean body mass, usually demonstrate less of a catabolic response to stress than men of comparable age and weight. Repeated stress will progressively erode the lean body mass, resulting in diminution of the quantity of nitrogen excreted with each catabolic episode. Nitrogen loss associated with intermittent fever from infection progressively decreases as nitrogen stores in the body are diminished.

4.22   HOW IS NITROGEN EXCRETION AFFECTED BY BED REST AND MUSCLE ACTIVITY?

Howard and associates[26] studied patients following operation and individuals with long-bone fractures and noted increased protein excretion in the trauma patients, averaging 190 g of protein per 1.73 m^2 body surface area. He also studied two normal men at bed rest who received 1600 kcal and 10 g of nitrogen per 1.73 m^2 body surface area, an adequate intake to achieve nitrogen equilibrium when not confined to bed. Negative nitrogen balance occurred in both volunteers with losses exceeding slightly more than 2 g/day in excess of intake.

Deitrick and co-workers studied the effects of immobilization on normal men placed in bivalved spica casts and maintained in bed for 6—7 weeks.[27] Nitrogen excretion increased on the 5—6th postimmobilization day and peaked during the first half of the second week

[25]Johnson, I. D.: The role of the endocrine glands on the metabolic response to operation. *Brit. J. Surg.* (Supp.), 54:438, 1967.

[26]Howard, J. E., Parson, W., Stein, K. E., Eisenberg, H., and Reidt, V.: Studies on fracture convalescence. I. Nitrogen metabolism after fracture and skeletal operation in healthy males. *Bull. Johns Hopkins Hosp.*, 75:156, 1944.

[27]Deitrick, J. E., Whedon, G. D., and Schorr, E.: Effects of immobilization upon various metabolic and physiologic functions of normal men. *Amer. J. Med.*, 4:3, 1948.

despite constant dietary intake that maintained nitrogen equilibrium during the control and recovery periods. Both urinary and fecal losses of calcium increased with immobilization and losses of sulfur, phosphorus, and potassium were also increased. In a subsequent study, three subjects were immobilized for 5 weeks but placed in oscillating beds.[28] Loss of nitrogen, calcium, and phosphorus was approximately half as great in patients in the oscillating bed when compared with similar studies in the fixed bed. In addition, most metabolic and physiologic functions returned to control levels or became restabilized more rapidly when the patients were treated in the oscillating beds. Physical therapy with isometric muscular contractions appears necessary to maintain lean body mass and cardio-circulatory tone appropriate for man's upright position.

4.23   HOW DOES STARVATION AFFECT NITROGEN EXCRETION FOLLOWING UNCOMPLICATED OPERATIONS? ... FOLLOWING COMPLICATED CASES OF INJURY AND INFECTION?

In patients undergoing small operations such as herniorrhaphy or elective intraabdominal procedures (cholecystectomy, gastrectomy), energy expenditure is unchanged, yet nitrogen balance is usually negative. Holden and Abbott studied patients following subtotal gastrectomy who were treated with varying intravenous caloric diets in the postoperative period.[29] Although none of the patients achieved positive nitrogen balance by the fourth postoperative day, there was a decrease in nitrogen loss with the administration of calories and nitrogen. This dose-related response significantly reduced loss of body nitrogen when compared to the postoperative patients receiving only 5% dextrose-containing solutions. The authors concluded that starvation played a significant role in the catabolic response following operation. In contrast, Howard could not achieve nitrogen balance following trauma by administering a high-protein diet during the peak of protein catabolism. However, nitrogen

[28]Whedon, G. D., Deitrick, J. E., and Shorr, E.: Modification of the effects of immobilization upon metabolic and physiologic functions of normal men by the use of an oscillating bed. *Amer. J. Med.*, 6:684, 1949.

[29]Holden, W. D., Krieger, H., Levey, S., and Abbott, W. E.: The effect of nutrition on nitrogen metabolism in the surgical patient. *Ann. Surg.*, 146:563, 1957.

Table 4.7   The Effect of Feeding on Nitrogen Loss Following Injury

Extent of injury	Nitrogen and caloric intake	Duration of negative nitrogen balance (days)	Cumulative negative nitrogen balance (g)
Minor trauma	None	3	24
Minor trauma	Constant intake[a]	2	3
Major trauma	None	10	90
Major trauma	Constant intake[a]	7	30

[a]10 g nitrogen/day.

Adapted from: Moore, F. D.: *Metabolic Care of the Surgical Patient*. Philadelphia, W. B. Saunders, 1959, p. 66.

equilibrium was maintained in a cachectic individual with long-bone fracture with moderate food intake.

Calorie and nitrogen intake diminishes or abates the post-traumatic negative nitrogen balance that occurs following injury (Table 4.7). While the quantity of nitrogen excreted increases in hypercatabolic patients following protein administration; negative nitrogen balance (intake − output) is appreciably diminished with food intake and nitrogen equilibrium may be achieved. Food intake exerts minimal effects on energy production (see Table 1.5, p. 16), and the specific dynamic action of ingested nutrients appears diminished in critically ill patients (p. 29).

4.24   IS THE NITROGEN LOSS FOLLOWING SEVERE INJURY THE RESULT OF DECREASED PROTEIN SYNTHESIS OR INCREASED PROTEIN BREAKDOWN?

Body protein stores are maintained by two opposing effects: protein synthesis and the rate of protein breakdown. In normal, fed individuals, these two rates are in equilibrium and the body's protein mass is maintained. During catabolic states, nitrogen loss from the body increases and this may be a result of decreased protein synthesis, increased protein breakdown, or a combination of both events. Studies in postoperative patients suggest that the catabolic response to operative stress involves a fall in protein synthesis without an associated increase in breakdown rates of body protein.[30] This

[30]O'Keefe, S. J. D., and Sender, P. M.: "Catabolic" loss of body nitrogen in response to surgery. *Lancet*, 2:1035, 1974.

alteration in amino acid dynamics occurred simultaneously with the increased excretion of urinary nitrogen. However, the patients studied were semistarved, and similar alterations in protein kinetics have been observed in individuals during food deprivation. Studies in severely injured and infected patients suggest that increased protein breakdown does occur; increased protein catabolism from muscle is supported by the exaggerated excretion of nitrogen lost in the urine following major trauma during zero nitrogen intake, the increase in creatinine and 3-methyl-histidine excretion suggesting muscle breakdown and the rapid wasting of the skeletal muscle mass.

4.25   WHAT ARE THE HORMONAL REGULATORS OF MUSCLE PROTEOLYSIS FOLLOWING INJURY AND INFECTION? HOW IS PROTEOLYSIS RELATED TO INCREASED UREAGENESIS?

Skeletal muscle breakdown is influenced by hormonal environment, passive and active contractions, and availability of nutrients. Insulin appears central to the regulation of protein metabolism and relative changes of plasma insulin levels are associated with muscle amino acid uptake or release.[31] Glucagon does not appear to have a peripheral effect on amino acid release but acts centrally on the liver.[32] Catecholamines stimulate an outpouring of lactic acid from muscle, and this is followed by an efflux of three-carbon amino acid fragments that shuttle carbon intermediates to the liver for conversion to new glucose. Glucocorticoids facilitate mobilization of amino acids which serve as glucose precursors. The new glucose may move back to the muscle and be converted to pyruvate in the cell. This three-carbon intermediate may receive an amino group from the branched-chain amino acids that are oxidized in muscle (Fig. 4.7). The new three-carbon nitrogen-containing compound, alanine, moves back to the liver with other three-carbon intermediates and is reconverted to new glucose; the nitrogen residue is simultaneously

[31] Brennan, M. F., Aoki, T. T., and Cahill, G. F., Jr.: Effect of insulin on glutamate uptake in the forearm muscles in postabsorptive state. Surg. Forum, 23:66, 1972.

[32] Fitzpatrick, G. F., Maguid, M. M., O'Connor, N. E., and Brennan, M. F.: Effects of glucagon on 3-methylhistidine excretion: Muscle proteolysis or ureogenesis? Surg. Forum, 26:46, 1975.

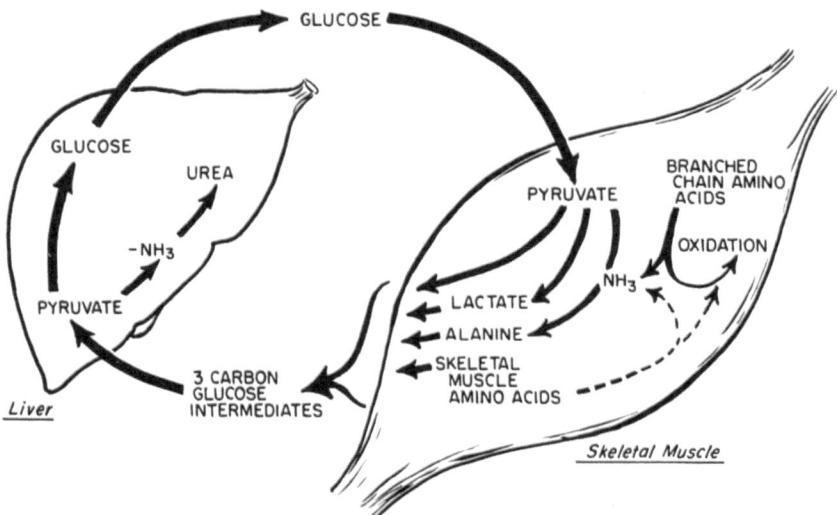

FIGURE 4.7: The increased elaboration of three-carbon intermediates from skeletal muscle provides glucose precursors for accelerated hepatic gluconeogenesis following infection or injury. The cycle as illustrated does not provide for the net loss of carbon from skeletal muscle, which is not representative of the decrease in muscle mass associated with catabolic diseases.

processed to urea. Thus, the rate of ureagenesis (reflected by urinary excretion of the urea) following stress generally correlates with the rate of gluconeogenesis.

4.26   WHAT DISEASE PROCESSES INCREASE METABOLIC RATE?

Increased basal metabolic rates occur with thyrotoxicosis, peritonitis, soft tissue or systemic infection, major trauma, and thermal injury (see p. 34). The increase in metabolism is related to the severity of injury or infection. Metabolic rate rarely exceeds twice normal levels in hospitalized disease-stressed patients, and this should be considered as the upper limit for heat production in critically ill patients supine in bed. Metabolic rate also varies with time postinjury, and oxygen consumption, which may be near normal during resuscitation, rises and peaks during the flow phase of injury and decreases in a curvilinear manner to return to predicted basal levels when wound healing or resolution of the infection is achieved (Fig. 4.6, p. 150). Cardiac output, ventilatory rate, and minute ventilation move parallel to the metabolic changes as if in response to the increased energy demands.

4.27   WHAT IS THE MEDIATOR OF THE INCREASED OXYGEN CONSUMPTION FOLLOWING INJURY?

The etiology of the hypermetabolic response following injury has been studied extensively, but the precise mechanisms have only recently been defined. Similarities between thermally injured patients and individuals with thyrotoxicosis prompted early endocrine studies by Oliver Cope and associates, but the increased oxygen consumption could not be associated with increased thyroid function.[33] Cuthbertson noted that the alterations in oxygen consumption were correlated with the increased excretion of nitrogen and suggested that the heat produced by protein catabolism and ureagenesis caused increased oxygen demand. Others, however, have not been able to account for the increased oxygen demand on the basis of this process of endogenous "specific dynamic activity."[34]

Catecholamines are elevated following injury, and adrenergic activity has been related to the severity of stress or extent of trauma and to oxygen consumption of the patient.[35] Carefully controlled adrenergic blockade in extensively injured patients consistently decreases metabolic rate, and infusion of epinephrine or norepinephrine in normal man increases metabolic rate. These studies demonstrate that increased sympathetic nervous system activity accounts for the increased heat production after injury and explains the similarity of response to a wide variety of stresses such as cold exposure, exercise, and infection.

Increased calorigenesis has also been noted with prolonged

[33]Cope, O., Nardi, G. L., Quijano, M., Rovit, R. L., Stanbury, J. B., and Wright, A.: Metabolic rate and thyroid function following acute thermal trauma in man. *Ann. Surg.,* *137*:165, 1953.

[34]Gusberg, R. J., Scholz, P. M., Gump, F. E., and Kinney, J. M.: Can protein breakdown explain the increased calorie expenditure in energy and sepsis? *Surg. Forum,* 24:79, 1973.

[35]Harrison, T. S., Seaton, J. F., and Feller, I.: Relationship of increased oxygen consumption to catecholamine excretion in thermal burns. *Ann. Surg.,* *165*:169, 1967.

growth hormone administration and infusion of glucagon.[36] The physiologic significance of these effects is yet to be determined, but these hormonal mediators may potentiate the catecholamine-mediated calorigenesis in injured man.

4.28 DOES EVAPORATIVE WATER LOSS FOLLOWING THERMAL INJURY CAUSE INCREASED HEAT PRODUCTION? WHAT IS THE ROLE OF ENVIRONMENTAL TEMPERATURE IN TREATING SEVERELY INJURED PATIENTS?

Increased oxygen consumption and insensible water loss are both correlated with burn size; hypermetabolism has previously been related to surface cooling secondary to increased evaporative water loss from the burn wound. Thermally injured patients treated in a warm environment ($32°C$) decrease metabolic rate, compared with treatment at $22°C$, and this evidence has been interpreted to support the thesis that hypermetabolism in burn patients is a response to increased surface cooling due to increased evaporative water loss. In contrast, Zawacki and associates covered the burn wound with a water-impermeable membrane (blocking evaporative water loss) but found no consistent alteration in metabolic rate in burn patients studied at approximately $25°C$ ambient temperature.[37]

Studies of burn patients in the rigidly controlled ambient conditions of an environmental chamber demonstrate that metabolism in normal subjects and patients with burns of less than 40% total body surface was not related to surface cooling by evaporative water loss. Hence, metabolic rate was unaffected when these individuals were studied at a warmer ambient temperature (Fig. 4.8). In patients with large thermal injuries, the decrease in dry heat loss exceeds the increase in wet heat loss in the $32°C$ environment, resulting in a consistent decrease in metabolic rate in patients with extensive thermal injury.

One of man's first defenses against cold exposure is to limit

[36]Aulick, H. L., Wilmore, D. W., and Mason, A. D., Jr.: Mechanism of glucagon calorigenesis. Fed. Proc., 35:401, 1976.
[37]Zawacki, B. E., Spitzer, K. W., Mason, A. D., Jr., and Johns, L. A.: Does increased evaporative water loss cause hypermetabolism in burned patients? Ann. Surg., 171:236, 1970.

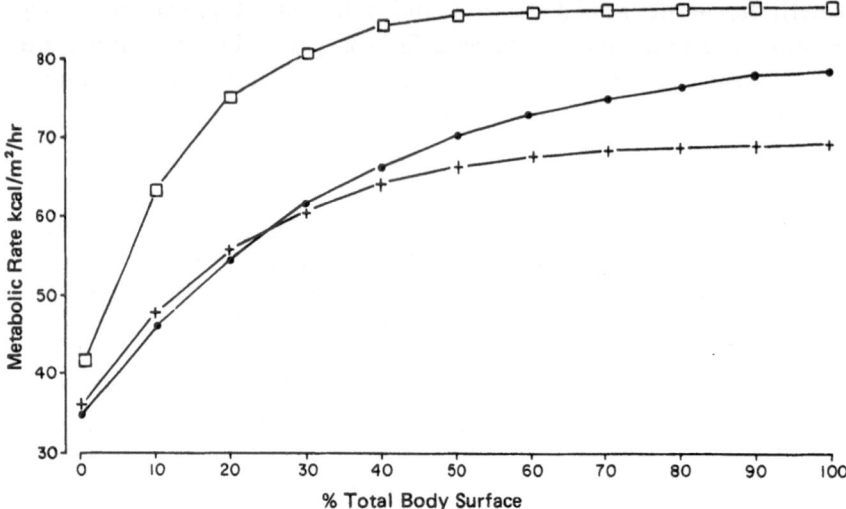

FIGURE 4.8: The predicted response of metabolic rate in burn patients and normals studied in three ambient environments with vapor pressure constant. The regression lines are described by the following equations where x = % total body surface burn and y = metabolic rate in kcal/m²/hr:

Ambient temperature	n	Relationship	r^2
21°C	12	$y = 86.84 - 45.48e^{-0.0673x}$	0.8997
25°C	22	$y = 81.29 - 46.63e^{-0.0286x}$	0.8821
33°C	21	$y = 69.84 - 34.82e^{-0.0457x}$	0.0819

□—□ 21°C, ●—● 25°C, +—+ 33°C.

evaporative water loss, but this is not accomplished in the burn patient because of damage to the surface. Another response to cold is to decrease the skin temperature and diminish dry heat loss. Both core and mean skin temperature were consistently 1.5–2.0°C higher in the thermally injured patients than in the controls. Core—skin heat conductivity (conductance, an index of superficial blood flow) increased with burn size: patients with large burns were characterized by inadequate core-to-skin insulation when exposed to cooler environments. Direct measurements of surface blood flow demonstrate that the increased flow is directed specifically to the wound, presumably to provide nutrients and increase tissue temperature, both processes essential for a rapid reparative process.

Evaporative water loss in burn patients is not the prime stimulator of the hypermetabolic response, but rather the increased energy production is related to an endogenous reset of metabolic activity. This basic metabolic drive is then influenced by environmental conditions. Metabolic rate does not return to normal levels with treatment of burn or severely injured patients in a warm environment, but metabolic activity can be minimized by caring for critically ill individuals in warm environments. Treatment of severely injured patients should be at temperatures which are generally above 28°C.

4.29 WHAT ALTERATIONS IN GLUCOSE DYNAMICS OCCUR FOLLOWING CRITICAL ILLNESS?

Hyperglycemia commonly occurs following injury and infection, and the elevation of fasting blood glucose above normal is generally related to the severity of the stress. Oral or intravenous glucose tolerance tests obtained from patients following hemorrhage or burn shock usually show a diabetic-like curve with prolonged disappearance of glucose from the blood stream and a persistent elevation of fasting glucose. Similar curves have been described in patients after elective operations and severe injury. Unfortunately these findings are difficult to interpret because of the partial starvation, bed rest, and inactivity which frequently accompanied early convalescence and injury. However, the tendency toward hyperglycemia and prolonged glucose intolerance has resulted in terms such as "traumatic diabetes" and "diabetes of injury," which generally suggest an insulin-deficient state, although hormonal response and glucose dynamics were not assessed. Moreover, the concept of insulin deficiency was appealing, for it explained in part the increased protein catabolism which occurs in critically ill patients. In contrast, Long and associates[38] demonstrated *increased* glucose flow through the extracellular fluid compartment in critically ill patients, and recent hepatic catheterization studies suggest that insulin inhibition of hepatic gluconeogenesis is dampened following injury.[39]

[38]Long, C. L., Spencer, J. L., Kinney, J. M., and Geiger, J. W.: Carbohydrate metabolism in man: Effect of elective operations and major injury. *J. Appl. Physiol., 31*:110, 1971.
[39]Gump, F. E., Long, C., Killian, P., and Kinney, J. M.: Studies of glucose intolerance in septic injured patients. *J. Trauma, 14*:378, 1974.

During the initial period of burn shock, serum glucose and body glucose (serum glucose x body glucose space) were elevated, and mass flow of glucose through the expanded glucose space (extracellular fluid compartment) was only slightly greater than normal (Table 4.8). The elevated body glucose appeared to be a function of the decreased instantaneous proportionality constant for glucose disappearance (k, see p. 96), which reflected impaired translocation of glucose into peripheral tissue. As the integrity of the extracellular fluid compartment was reestablished and normal circulation was achieved following resuscitation, the patients moved from the "ebb" phase of injury to the "flow" phase. At this point in time (6–16 days postinjury), the rate of glucose disappearance was enhanced. The proportionality constant for glucose disappearance was similar to that obtained in normal individuals in spite of a persistent hyperglycemia which was observed in the burn patients. Glucose flow was significantly elevated in the burn patients compared to normal individuals, suggesting that the increase in blood glucose observed in these individuals is a consequence of increased hepatic production of glucose, not altered peripheral disappearance, as determined by the instantaneous proportionality constant for glucose disappearance. Glucose flow was related to the extent of injury and returned to normal with closure of the burn wound.

4.30 HOW DOES THE INSULIN RESPONSE VARY DURING THE ACUTE AND HYPERMETABOLIC PHASES OF INJURY?

Fasting serum insulin levels were comparable in the normals, the patients with burn shock, and in the individuals studied during the hypermetabolic phase (Table 4.8), but insulin levels were significantly diminished in the resuscitated patients when basal insulin was expressed as the ratio of its absolute value to fasting blood glucose. As previously reported by Allison, Hinton, and Chamberlain,[40] the insulin response during burn shock resuscitation was significantly blunted. Following burn shock resuscitation, the insulin response to injected glucose appeared comparable in burn patients (6–16 days)

[40]Allison, S. P., Hinton, P., and Chamberlain, M. J.: Intravenous glucose tolerance, insulin, and free-fatty-acid levels in burned patients. *Lancet*, 2:1113, 1968.

Table 4.8 Glucose Dynamics Following Injury

	N	Fasting serum glucose (mg/100 ml)	Glucose space (liters/kg)	Body glucose (mg/kg)	k (100 min^{-1})	Glucose flow $\dot{Q}$ (mg/kg/min)	Basal insulin (μU/ml)	Insulinogenic index
Controls	12	70 ± 2	0.152 ± 0.010	106 ± 5	4.01 ± 0.56	3.29 ± 0.32	22 ± 3	0.48 ± 0.10
Burn shock resuscitation	4	140 ± 11	0.349 ± 0.010	483 ± 22	1.21 ± 0.12	5.81 ± 0.44	20 ± 6	0.21 ± 0.07
Burns (6–16 days)	17	113 ± 5	0.117 ± 0.010	200 ± 11	5.27 ± 0.51	10.12 ± 0.95	22 ± 2	0.52 ± 0.07
Septic burn patients	15	116 ± 10	0.220 ± 0.015	255 ± 29	2.62 ± 0.47	5.66 ± 0.80	22 ± 4	0.24 ± 0.04
Burn patients, previous sepsis	4	110 ± 15	0.233 ± 0.010	258 ± 25	1.80 ± 0.54	4.56 ± 1.67	12 ± 3	0.10 ± 0.03

when compared to normals (insulinogenic index described on p. 93).

These observations are consistent with present knowledge of adrenergic control of the beta pancreatic cell, for alpha-receptor stimulation inhibits insulin release and beta-receptor stimulation augments insulin elaboration. During burn shock resuscitation, the alpha receptor inhibitory effect appears dominant, insulin output is decreased, and diabetic-like glucose tolerance curves are observed. As the burn patient becomes hypermetabolic in the second week postinjury, profound beta-adrenergic receptor stimulatory effects are observed, characterized by increased basal heat production. At this time, normal concentrations of fasting insulin and an appropriate insulin response to glucose load are observed; glucagon concentrations are elevated. Subtle adjustments in the sympathetic nervous system reflect these alterations in metabolic control, with both alpha- and beta-adrenergic receptor effects observed in the "ebb" phase of injury (afferent stimuli during the shock phase may be hypovolemia, hypoxia, acidosis, or pain), while beta-receptor effects dominate during the hypermetabolic or "flow" phase.

The instantaneous proportionality constant for glucose disappearance was related to the insulin response as previously described in normals and diabetic patients (Fig. 3.4, p. 98). The proportionality constant for glucose disappearance was not related to fasting insulin levels but was associated with the early or total insulin response (0—10 insulinogenic index or total insulinogenic index).

4.31   WHAT IS THE REGULATOR OF HEPATIC GLUCONEOGENESIS?

As previously noted, hepatic gluconeogenesis is directed by an interaction of hormones; insulin favors hepatic glucose storage, and catecholamines, augmented by glucagon and glucocorticoids, signal for hepatic glucose production. The increased sympathetic activity directs the response of the endocrine pancreatic hormones following stress, and insulin and glucagon, in turn, regulate the disposition of key substrates under their control. Mobilization of substrate from the periphery is stimulated by catecholamines augmented by glucocorticoids, and this "signal for mobilization" is increased with insulin

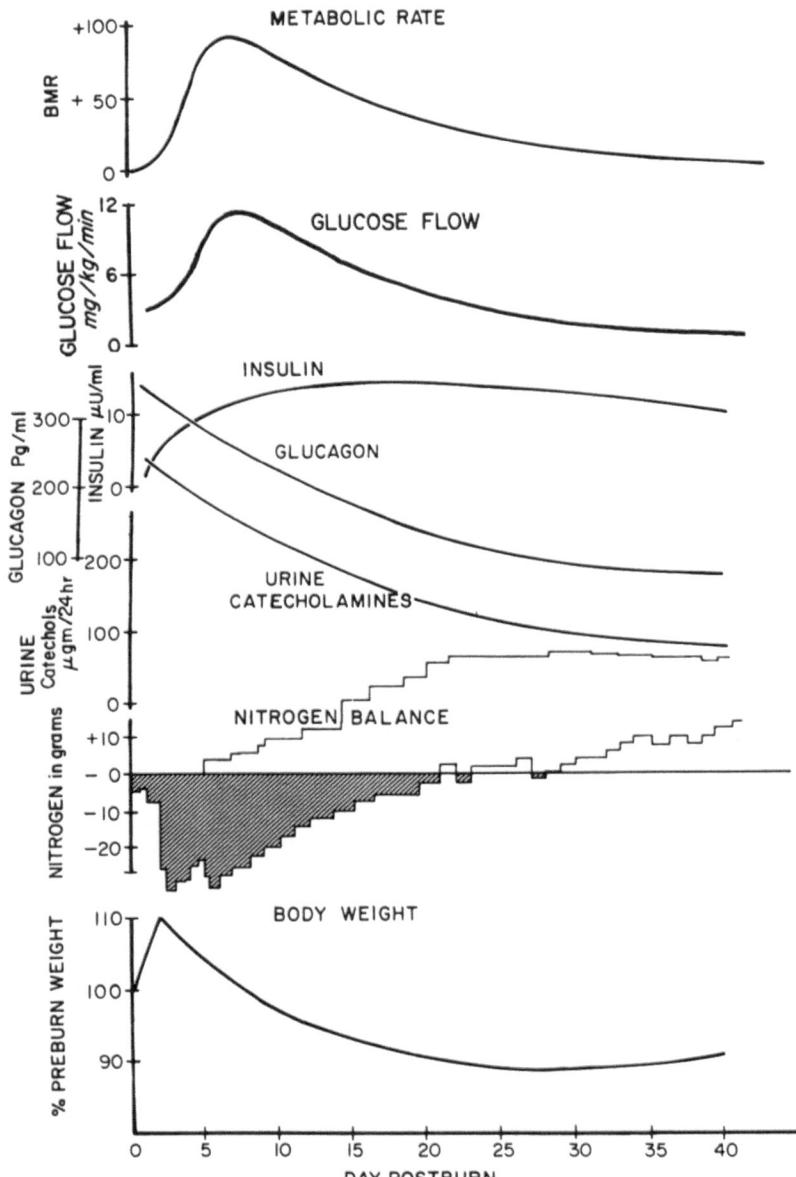

FIGURE 4.9: The increased rate of hepatic glucose production (glucose flow) parallels the hypermetabolic response following thermal injury. Increased gluconeogenesis is associated in time with negative nitrogen balance and high levels of glucagon and catecholamines relative to insulin. As these hormonal mediators return to normal, oxygen consumption and hepatic glucose production fall and nitrogen balance becomes positive.

deficiency. Thus, increased adrenergic activity appears as the major mediator of the metabolic response following injury or infection, regulating substrate mobilization, controlling substrate cycling (through the Cori and alanine cycles), and stimulating hepatic gluconeogenesis (Fig. 4.9).

4.32 WHAT ALTERATIONS IN GLUCOSE DYNAMICS OCCUR DURING CONVALESCENCE?

Glucose dynamics in convalescent patients following severe injury are similar to findings of glucose kinetics in starved or semistarved man. With progressive resolution of the injury, serum glucose and the proportionality constant for glucose disappearance decreased. The decrease of k was associated with a diminution of fasting insulin levels and a decrease in insulin response to a glucose load (Table 4.9). These alterations were associated in time with a decrease in body weight of approximately 11%.

Table 4.9   Five Patients Studied before and after Closure of the Burn Wound (Mean ± SE, Range)

	Early	Late
Postburn day studied	13 ± 2 (7—18)	69 ± 9 (37—90)
Body weight (kg)	60.2 ± 4.8 (43.3—72.0)	53.3 ± 3.2[a] (40.9—58.7)
Fasting glucose (mg/100 ml)	116 ± 4 (106—126)	73 ± 6[b] (55—85)
k (100 min^{-1})	4.51 ± 0.68 (2.92—6.90)	1.99 ± 0.20[a] (1.29—2.47)
Fasting insulin (μU/ml)	29 ± 6 (18—46)	14 ± 1 (9—16)
Insulinogenic index	0.39 ± 0.07 (0.19—0.60)	0.22 ± 0.01[a] (0.18—0.25)

[a] $p < 0.05$.   [b] $p < 0.01$.

4.33 HOW ARE GLUCOSE DYNAMICS ALTERED WITH INFECTION? WITH GRAM-NEGATIVE SEPSIS COMPLICATING INJURY?

Hepatic glucose production increases with bacterial infection in man, and the increased rate of gluconeogenesis is generally related to the extent of infection. In contrast, gram-negative infection or endotoxin administration to animals blocks hepatic gluconeogenesis, depletes glycogen stores, and causes a progressive fall in blood glucose concentrations.[41] Hypoglycemia has occasionally been observed in man, and is most commonly observed in the neonate with gram-negative infection.[42]

In patients with extensive injury, glucose flow and hepatic glucose production are increased, but decrease toward normal during periods of gram-negative bacteremia (Table 4.8). Gluconeogenic precursors increase in concentration in the blood stream and alanine administration fails to cause a rise in serum glucose in injured patients with gram-negative bacteremia.[43] Increased hepatic glucose production can be augmented with glucagon infusion (but not insulin administration), supporting the thesis that the liver is the primary site of decreased gluconeogenesis. Animal studies suggest that this effect is mediated by endotoxin, which blocks glycogen formation and interferes with alanine, pyruvate, and lactate conversion to glucose. In injured man, the decreased hepatic production of glucose appears to persist after the blood stream is cleared of infection, suggesting that sustained impairment of hepatic function may occur following endotoxemia.

4.34 HOW IS HEAT PRODUCTION RELATED TO INCREASED GLUCOSE FLOW? IS THE INCREASED GLUCOSE FLOW NECESSARY TO PROVIDE AN OXIDIZED FUEL?

Increased flow of glucose from the liver to the periphery occurs during the hypermetabolic, reparative, or flow phase of injury. The glucose appears to be converted to three-carbon intermediates which return to the liver for resynthesis to new glucose, utilizing metabolic pathways described by the Cori cycle and alanine shuttle system (Fig. 4.10). Entry of glucose into the tricarboxylic acid cycle is limited, a finding consistent with earlier studies which suggest a partial block in metabolic pathways leading from three-carbon to

[41] LaNoue, K. F., Mason, A. D., Jr., and Daniels, J. P.: The impairment of glucogenesis by gram negative infection. *Metabolism, 17*:606, 1968.

[42] Yeung, C. Y.: Hypoglycemia in neonatal sepsis. *J. Pediatr., 77*:812, 1970.

[43] Wilmore, D. W., Mason, A. D., Jr., and Pruitt, B. A. Jr.: Impaired glucose flow in burned patients with gram-negative sepsis. *Surg. Gynecol. Obstet., 143*:720, 1976.

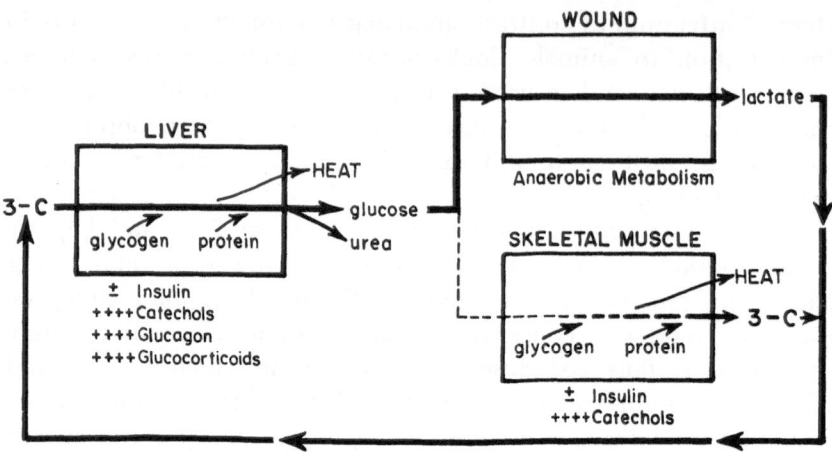

FIGURE 4.10: The flow of six- and three-carbon units following injury is increased. Heat production is related to rate of six-carbon—three-carbon flow. Anaerobic metabolism in the wound contributes lactate to the three-carbon pool while both lactate and amino acid may arise from skeletal muscle. Studies in noninfected injured patients demonstrate that the major glucose flow is to the wound. Not shown is the three-carbon contribution of glycerol from body fat.

two-carbon fragments following operative injury.[44] Enzymes which favor conversion of three-carbon intermediates to glucose are pyruvate carboxylase and phosphoenolpyruvate carboxylase; increased synthesis of these enzymes occurs in the presence of high levels of glucocorticoids, glucagon, and catecholamines, and low levels of insulin, precisely the hormone environment present during the catabolic phase of injury (Fig. 4.11).

Both heat production and glucose flow increase with the extent of injury, and these two factors also appear to change together with time following injury (Fig. 4.9). Simultaneous measurements of glucose flow and oxygen consumption demonstrate a close relationship between the mass flow of glucose through the extracellular compartment and heat production (Fig. 4.12). However, this relationship did not occur because glucose was oxidized as a primary fuel source; in contrast, all the respiratory quotients of these patients studied were low (0.70–0.75), reflecting the oxidation of fat as the primary fuel substrate.

[44]Drucker, W. R., Craig, J., Kingsbury, B., Hofmann, N., and Woodward, H.: Citrate metabolism during surgery. *Arch. Surg., 85:*557, 1962.

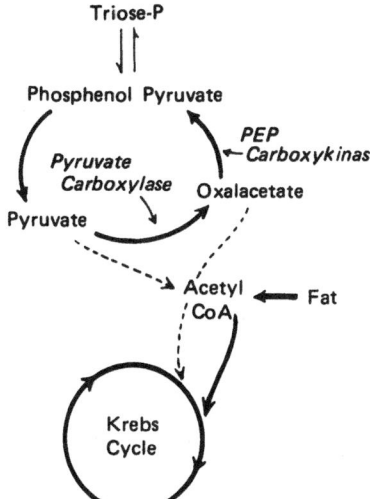

FIGURE 4.11: Three-carbon—two-carbon interaction in cycling. Entry of glucose via pyruvate into the Krebs cycle is limited because of an endocrine environment which induces enzymes favoring conversion of three-carbon intermediates to glucose.

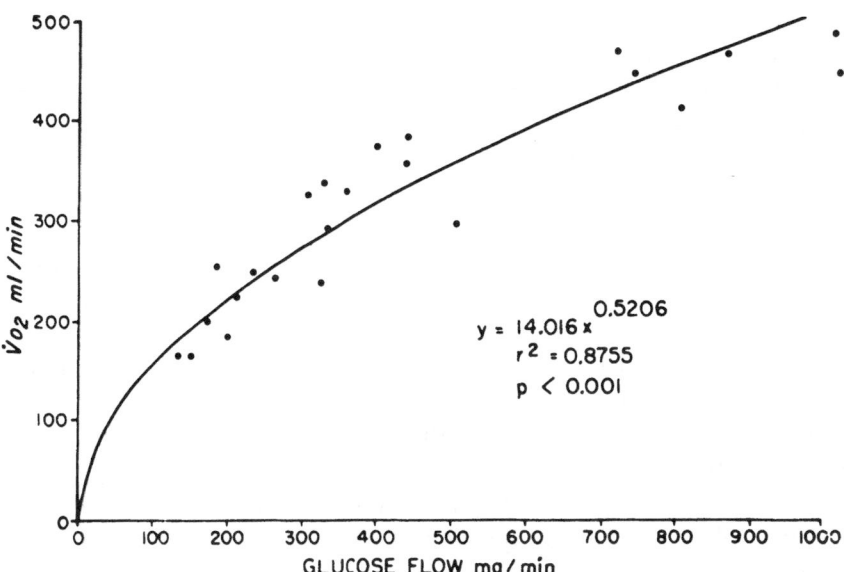

FIGURE 4.12: Oxygen consumption is related with mass flow of glucose in extensively injured patients.

Finally, the biochemical processing of three-carbon intermediates and glucose is a heat-producing reaction. Stimulation of gluconeogenesis with glucagon infusion in normal man produces a dose-response increase in oxygen consumption. The increased heat production was accompanied by a rise in blood glucose, insulin, and respiratory quotient, all indicating increased flow of glucose to peripheral tissues. However, the increased heat production could not be duplicated by the glucose infusion alone. Similarly, gram-negative bacteremia in extensively injured man causes a decrease in glucose production and a simultaneous fall in heat production.

4.35   WHAT TISSUE COMPONENTS OF THE BODY ARE ASSOCIATED WITH WEIGHT LOSS FOLLOWING INJURY OR INFECTION? IS POSTINJURY WEIGHT LOSS OBLIGATORY?

Most easily recognized and readily documented is the loss of body weight which occurs after injury or during infection. Like other metabolic responses, weight loss is related to the extent of stress: the greater the stress, the greater the weight loss. Moore interpreted studies of body composition as indicating that cellular loss was approximately half fat and half lean body mass following severe surgical stress. Duke and associates noted that the ratio of fuel burned in stressed patients was remarkably constant, with fat contributing 80–85% of the calories utilized and the remaining energy originating from body protein. In addition, a large component of weight loss is water, and weight loss or weight stabilization in the surgical patient is often a reflection of loss or gain in total body water.

Weight loss after injury is not an obligatory component of the response to trauma, but rather reflects the difference between energy requirements of the patient and the ability to provide these requirements in the form of adequate calories. Recent developments in feeding techniques allow vigorous enteral–parenteral nutritional support following injury, replacing or exceeding caloric and nitrogen requirements in the stressed patients. Weight loss can be diminished or essentially prevented if energy support equals energy demand. Although feeding the patient does not alter the autonomic nervous system response to injury, calorie and nitrogen intake minimizes or prevents severe protein wasting which may in itself alter body function.

4.36 WHAT ALTERATIONS IN INTERMEDIARY METABOLISM OCCUR DURING EXERCISE? HOW DOES THIS RESPONSE DIFFER FROM THE CHANGES WHICH OCCUR IN CRITICALLY INJURED MAN?

The increased oxygen consumption occurs primarily in the working muscle; heat production increases proportionally with the extent of exercise. Maximum oxygen consumption with exercise is 10–15 times greater than basal metabolic rates. In contrast, injured or infected patients in bed seldom exceed more than twice the normal basal levels of heat production. Glycogen stores in the muscle are rapidly utilized and hepatic gluconeogenesis maintains the arterial glucose concentration; skeletal muscle utilization of glucose may exceed hepatic glucose production and serum glucose concentrations fall. Free fatty acids contribute a large proportion of the oxidized fuel for muscle as time progresses. Muscle output of lactate, pyruvate, and alanine increases and these three-carbon fragments account for an increasing proportion of the precursors of the hepatic glucose produced.[45] Blood flow to skeletal muscle increases in response to metabolic demands of exercise; this increased peripheral blood flow is associated with a decrease in splanchnic blood flow. Unlike an injured man, a runner can stop to rest, and body-fuel stores and substrate turnover return to normal during the recovery period.

4.37 WHAT ALTERATIONS IN INTERMEDIARY METABOLISM OCCUR WITH COLD EXPOSURE?

When exposed to cold, man increases his metabolic rate to produce more heat, maintain heat balance, and stabilize core temperature. During the initial period of cold exposure, shivering is the major mechanism of heat production. This response can be blunted or

[45] Ahlborg, G., Felig, P., Hagenfeldt, L., Hendler, R., and Wahren, J.: Substrate turnover during prolonged exercise in man. *J. Clin. Invest., 53*:1080, 1974.

abolished in small animals exposed to cold by administration of curare, resulting in a rapid fall in body temperature. Although shivering is an effective mechanism of heat production, it is not efficient for maintenance of body temperature. The gross movements of shivering actually increase environmental heat loss and interfere with skilled movements and sleep.

Shivering causes skeletal muscle contraction, which increases the rate of hydrolysis of ATP to ADP by the muscle cell; no net mechanical work results, and the free energy released by ATP hydrolysis is converted to heat. ADP concentration regulates electron transport and oxygen consumption, a process referred to as "receptor control." In a response similar to that during exercise, carbohydrate and fat are the primary fuels utilized by the muscle mass during acute cold exposure. Substrate cycling to the liver also occurs.

With long-term cold exposure, cold acclimatization occurs, allowing the organism to respond to a cold ambient environment more rapidly and efficiently.

CHAPTER 5

Feeding the Patient

5.1 HAS VIGOROUS NUTRITIONAL SUPPORT ALWAYS BEEN PROVIDED TO CRITICALLY ILL PATIENTS? WHAT EVIDENCE SUGGESTS THAT IT IS ESSENTIAL TO PATIENT CARE?

Starvation was the accepted practice for centuries in patients with fever, and this treatment frequently included water deprivation. Graves suggested that the deleterious effects of starvation compounded the consequences of disease, and recommended a diet for patients with hypermetabolism secondary to infection and thyrotoxicosis that was considered revolutionary for the times.[1] Although the nutritional intake consisted of only sugar water, meat broths, toast crumbs, and jellies, and probably provided no more than 300 kcal/day, this meager oral diet therapy became the accepted means of nutritional support of the day. Graves was convinced of the value of nutrition for critically ill patients, and late in life, suggested that his own epitaph read "He Feeds Fever." In the late 1800s, a milk diet for typhoid fever was proposed, and later, Peabody advocated the more liberal use of standard oral feedings. However, it was not until the classic studies of Coleman and DuBois in the early 1900s, that nutritional management of the critically ill patient was based on a firm foundation of scientific fact.[2] They concluded that (1) body fuels are oxidized to the same end-products as in health, and the laws of the conservation of energy apply to fever patients; (2) the specific dynamic action of protein and carbohydrate is much smaller in the febrile patient with typhoid fever than in the healthy individual; and (3) increased breakdown of protein occurs in infected patients, and the negative nitrogen balance could not be offset by positive energy balance at the levels of protein intake that were utilized (approximately 15 g of nitrogen per day).

The specific dietary requirement suggested by Coleman was food equivalent to 4000 kcal/day in a 150-lb man.[3] The diet was high in carbohydrate and protein, based on the studies that demonstrated "carbohydrate protects body protein better than any other foodstuff," and nutrients were provided by meals and interval

[1] Graves, R. J.: *Lectures on the Practice of Medicine.* Dublin, New Sydenham Society, 1884.
[2] Coleman, W., and DuBois, E. F.: Clinical calorimetry. VII Calorimetric observations on the metabolism of typhoid patients with and without food. *Ann. Int. Med., 15:*887, 1915.
[3] Coleman, W.: Diet in typhoid fever. *J. Am. Med. Assoc., 53:*1145, 1909.

feedings. Thus, it became accepted that partial starvation was detrimental to the patient's welfare. It was "not only desirable but necessary" that the typhoid patient be given sufficient exogenous nutrients to equal energy expenditure.

While the body's catabolic response to injury and infection could be offset by high-calorie, high-nitrogen feedings, techniques of nutrient delivery and product availability remained the single deterrent for providing adequate nutritional support for the critically ill, hospitalized patient. This final hurdle was overcome by the development of a technique for central venous cannulation and infusion of hypertonic nutrient solutions, the formulation and evolution of techniques for administration of defined bulk-free formula enteral diets, and the development of a safe fat emulsion for intravenous administration.

5.2 HOW PREVALENT IS HOSPITAL MALNUTRITION? WHY DOES IT OCCUR?

Protein—calorie malnutrition is most frequently seen in this country in hospitalized patients. Nutritional surveys of individuals admitted to both medical and surgical services reveal that 25—50% of the patients in large hospitals demonstrate unequivocal signs of protein—calorie malnutrition.[4,5]

Butterworth suggests that the nutritional problem is most often iatrogenic, occurring because of the failure of physicians to concern themselves with nutritional needs of the patients, while practicing sophisticated and highly advanced medical care and performing extensive operative procedures.[6] He attributes the poor nutritional health of hospitalized patients to the following undesirable practices:

1. Failure to record the admission height and weight of a patient and failure to accurately weigh the patient while in the hospital.
2. Rotation of the hospital staff and diffusion of responsibility for the patient's nutritional care.
3. Withholding meals for diagnostic tests.

[4]Butterworth, C. E., Jr.: Malnutrition in the hospital. *J. Am. Med. Assoc.*, 230:879, 1974.
[5]Bistrian, B. R., Blackburn, G. L., Hallowell, E., and Hadelle, R.: Protein status of general surgical patients. *J. Am. Med. Assoc.*, 230:858, 1974.
[6]Butterworth, C. E., Jr.: The skeleton in the hospital closet. *Nutrition Today*, 9:4, 1974.

4. Inability to assess nutritional deficiencies when the patient enters the hospital and failure to determine nutritional requirements of various disease processes.
5. Delay of nutritional support until the patient is in an advanced state of nutritional depletion.
6. Lack of appreciation of the role of adequate nutrition in the prevention, treatment, and resolution of many diseases. In particular, an overreliance on the use of antibiotics to treat infection, administration of chemotherapy to the cancer patient in the face of starvation, and treatment of the patient with trauma or gastrointestinal dysfunction without regard for nutritional intake.

5.3   HOW DOES MALNUTRITION IMPAIR THE PATIENT'S RESPONSE TO DISEASE?

The physiological effects of starvation have been previously reviewed (see p. 142). However, several major alterations which are frequently associated with malnutrition occur in critically ill patients and may impair the optimal homeostatic response to disease.[7] Hypoproteinemia is frequently observed in nutritionally depleted patients, but is also observed in well-nourished individuals with sequestration of albumin at the site of extensive operative dissection, inflammation, or injury. The hypoproteinemic patient is extremely susceptible to excess intake of salt and/or water; edema may form in the visceral tissues as well as in the extremities. Visceral edema has been associated with prolonged gastric emptying, enterostomy malfunction, and delayed intestinal transit time. Wound edema interferes with healing, and the restoration of serum oncotic pressure restores the rate of fibroplasia to normal. Finally, animals rendered hypoproteinemic by plasmapheresis could withstand only 60% of the blood volume deficit following controlled hemorrhage as normal animals, suggesting that hypoproteinemia increases the organism's susceptibility to shock.

[7] Rhoads, J. E.: Nutrition. *In* Rhoads, J. E., Allen, J. G., Harkins, H. N., and Moyer, C. A. (Eds.): *Surgery: Principals and Practice*, 4th Ed., Philadelphia, J. B. Lippincott, 1970, p. 101.

With progressive malnutrition, there is decreased strength and activity. Wasting of the musculature involved with respiration compromises pulmonary function and results in inefficient ventilation. Inactivity increases the risk of thrombophlebitis and decubitus ulcers. Bed rest and lack of exercise progressively decondition the cardiovascular system to the upright position.

Wound healing and resolution of inflammation depend on the availability of basic nutrients for phagocytic function and tissue repair. Hypovolemia, anemia, and wound edema may interfere with transport of nutrients to the wound; low wound oxygen tension and a decreased wound pH result. When these transport factors are corrected, essential substrate then becomes rate-limiting; glucose, amino acids, vitamins, and trace elements are essential for normal fibroplasia and epithelialization.

The susceptibility of the malnourished patient to infection is well known. The deficiency in host resistance is additive to immunological defects associated with various disease processes. Exposure to infection is more frequent in critically ill patients with multiple indwelling catheters, nasotracheal tubes, and breaks in skin or other membrane barriers. In addition, use of steroids and antibiotics may favor proliferation of opportunistic organisms which are poised to invade the malnourished immunologically deficient host.

The risk of a standard operative procedure in a nutritionally depleted patient is increased,[8] and a previously healthy individual's ability to withstand a prolonged illness is compromised if adequate nutritional support is not provided.

5.4   HOW IS THE EXTENT OF MALNUTRITION OR STARVATION BEST QUANTITATED IN MAN?

Although an adequate history, including a review of daily food intake, and careful physical examination aid the physician in diagnosing specific nutritional deficiencies (Table 5.1), it may be difficult to quantitate the extent of protein—calorie malnutrition in

---

[8]Studley, H. O.: Percentage of weight loss: A basic indicator of surgical risk in patients with chronic peptic ulcer. *J. Amer. Med. Assoc., 106*:458, 1936.

Table 5.1   Some Clinical Signs of Probable Nutritional Significance

Hair	Lack of luster Easy pluckability	Tongue	Edema Glossitis Magenta tongue
Skin	Follicular hyperkeratosis Petechiae, purpura Pellagrous dermatitis Scrotal and vulval dermatitis	Gums	Swollen interdental papillae Bleeding
		Teeth	Mottled enamel
Face	Nasolabial seborrhea	Glands	Thyroid enlargement Parotid enlargement
Eyes	Xerosis of conjunctivae Keratomalacia Corneal vascularization Circumcorneal injection Blepharitis Photophobia Bitot's spots	Skeleton	Enlarged wrist epiphysis Bossing of the skull Beading of the ribs Bowed legs
		Neurological	Absent vibratory sense in the feet Hyporeflexia Decreased position sense Tender calf muscles
Lips	Cheilosis Bilateral angular fissures Bilateral angular scars	Extremities	Dependent edema

Adapted from: Sandstead, H. H. and Pearson, W. N.: Clinical evaluation of nutritional status. *In* Goodhart, R. S. and Shils, M. E. (Eds.): *Modern Nutrition in Health and Disease*, 5th ed., 1973, Philadelphia, Lea and Febiger, p. 581.

specific patients and/or to adequately assess the impact of nutritional therapy. Several objective criteria may be utilized to determine the nutritional status of the patient:

1. Body weight and rate of weight loss (p. 50): As previously noted, weight loss of more than 10% or a recent rapid weight loss of up to 6% body weight indicates that further nutritional evaluation of the patient is necessary. Appropriate nutritional therapy should be instituted.

2. Anthropometric measurements: Triceps skin fold thickness and arm muscle circumference correlate reasonably well with body composition.[9] Girth and thigh measurements may also be taken, but all these dimensions are only reliable when obtained by experienced observers. Variations in height, weight, extent of

[9]Jelliffe, D. B.: *The Assessment of the Nutritional Status of the Community*. World Health Organization, 1966.

obesity, sex, age, and the presence of edema contribute to error in these measurements.

3. Body compositional measurements: A reliable laboratory is necessary for accurate determination of body composition; total body potassium, which is related to the size of the lean-body mass, is measured by isotope dilution technique or by whole-body counter. Determination of total body water or body density (using immersion techniques) allows estimation of body fat mass. Other assessments of body composition are available.[10]

4. Creatinine—height ratio: Twenty-four-hour creatinine excretion is related to the size of the muscle mass. This value is adjusted for height to quantify depletion of muscle mass in adults.[11]

5. Tests of immune function: Total peripheral lymphocyte count, response to skin tests, and lymphocyte transformation to mitogens are reliable indicators of immunocompetence of the patients. These tests of immune function often show depressed values in malnourished patients and return toward normal with nutritional repletion.[12]

6. Blood analysis: Hemoglobin and red blood cell indices, serum albumin and total protein concentration, serum amino acid profiles and acute-phase protein concentration (transferrin or iron binding capacity and others) are useful (Table 5.2). Serum vitamin and trace element concentrations may document specific deficiencies.

5.5 WHAT ARE THE INDICATIONS FOR VIGOROUS NUTRITIONAL SUPPORT OF HOSPITALIZED PATIENTS?

The day is past when adequate nutrition cannot be provided to all hospitalized patients. No longer should protein—calorie malnutrition be an additive stress to the individual with a catabolic disease process. Nutritional support of all patients should become a planned and integral part of therapy and not an afterthought. In the critically

[10]Moore, F. D.: *The Body Cell Mass and Its Supporting Environment.* Philadelphia, W. B. Saunders, 1963.

[11]Bistrian, B. R., Blackburn, G. L., Sherman, M., and Scrimshaw, N. S.: Therapeutic index of nutritional depletion in hospitalized patients. *Surg. Gynecol. Obstet., 141*:512, 1975.

[12]Law, D. K., Dudrick, S. J., and Abdou, N. I.: The effects of protein calorie malnutrition on immune competence of the surgical patient. *Surg. Gynecol. Obstet., 139*:257, 1974.

Table 5.2   Suggested Guide for Interpreting Blood Concentrations
(from the National Nutritional Survey)

	Deficient	Low	Acceptable
Hemoglobin (g/100 ml)			
Men	< 12.0	12.0–13.9	⩾14.0
Women[a]	< 10.0	10.0–11.9	⩾12.0
Children (2–5 yrs)	< 10.0	10.0–10.9	⩾11.0
Children (6–12 yrs)	< 10.0	10.0–11.4	⩾11.5
Hemoglobin concentration (MCHC) (g/100 ml RBC)			
For all ages and sex		30	⩾30
Serum iron (μg/100 ml)			
Men		<60	⩾60
Women[a]		<40	⩾40
Children (2–5 yrs)		<40	⩾40
Children (6–12 yrs)		<50	⩾50
Transferrin saturation (%)			
Men		<20	⩾20
Women[a]		<15	⩾15
Children (2–5 yrs)		<20	⩾20
Children (6–12 yrs)		<20	⩾20
Red cell folacin (mμg/ml)			
All ages	<140	140–159	⩾160–650
Serum folacin (mμg/ml)			
All ages	< 3.0	3.0–5.9	> 6.0
Serum albumin (g/100 ml)			
Adults	< 2.8	2.8–3.4	> 3.5
Children (1–5 yrs)		< 3.0	> 3.0
Children (6–17 yrs)		< 3.5	> 3.5
Serum ascorbic acid (mg/100 ml)			
All ages	< 0.1	0.1–0.19	> 0.2
Plasma carotene (μg/100 ml)			
Adult[a]		<40	⩾40
Children (1–17 yrs)		<40	⩾40
Plasma vitamin A (μg/100 ml)			
All ages	< 10	10–19	⩾20

[a]Nonpregnant, nonlactating.

ill patient, other priorities of care should be attended to before some
of the more complex techniques of nutritional support are initiated.
These include adequate oxygenation and tissue perfusion, normal
hydration and electrolyte balance, and restoration of blood volume.
In addition, the factors of cost and risk in a specific hospital setting
must be balanced against known nutritional gains in a particular
patient with a specific disease process before some forms of

nutritional therapy are initiated. All of these considerations are part of the equation which predicts which nutritional therapy to institute and at what point in time a specific dietary program should be altered.

Three factors determine the *quantity* of energy to be administered: (1) the nutritional state of the patient; (2) the extent of catabolism associated with a specific disease process; and (3) the time that has elapsed from the onset of a disease process. A patient with a normal body mass without a hypercatabolic illness can easily sustain normal physiological function for days before nutritional factors contribute to altered homeostasis. If weight loss is greater than 10% of normal predicted body weight, malnutrition will interact with a disease process to impair host responses; vigorous restoration of nutritional balance should be instituted. Similarly, a moderately depleted individual admitted to the hospital with a hypercatabolic disease process should not be subjected to ongoing malnutrition. Vigorous nutritional support, by whatever route possible, should be provided (Fig. 5.1).

With time, following the onset of a disease, the quantity of energy required for maintenance and/or restoration of the body cell mass may change. More vigorous nutritional support is usually required. The safest and most effective route of nutrient administration should be utilized to provide the increased nutrient requirements. Although the risks may increase utilizing tube feeding techniques or parenteral nutrient infusions, complication rates have been minimized in many institutions by training personnel who supervise the nutritional support techniques. If resources are not available or an appropriate protocol which minimizes the hazards of nutritional support cannot be followed in a particular institution, referral of the patient to a center with nutritional support capabilities should be considered early in the individual's hospital course. Many new techniques utilize modified diets designed to achieve optimal nutrition during a specific disease process in a specific category of patients. Such highly sophisticated nutritional support requires a multidisciplinary team for effective and safe delivery. The "nutritional urgency" for patient referral is not as apparent as in individuals with refractory cardiovascular failure or acute renal failure if the physician is not aware of the importance nutritional support plays in many of the lethal diseases observed in hospitalized patients today.

5.6 WHAT ARE THE BEST RECOMMENDATIONS AVAILABLE FOR

Recommended Daily Dietary Allowances, Revised 1974, Food and Nutrition
the maintenance of good nutrition of practically all healthy people in the USA)

							Fat-soluble vitamins				
	Age (years)	Weight (kg)	(lb)	Height (cm)	(in)	Energy (kcal)[b]	Protein (g)	Vitamin A Activity (RE)[c]	(IU)	Vitamin D (IU)	Vitamin E Activity[e] (IU)	Ascorbic Acid (mg)
Infants	0.0–0.5	6	14	60	24	kg × 117	kg × 2.2	420[d]	1,400	400	4	35
	0.5–1.0	9	20	71	28	kg × 108	kg × 2.0	400	2,000	400	5	35
Children	1–3	13	28	86	34	1300	23	400	2,000	400	7	40
	4–6	20	44	110	44	1800	30	500	2,500	400	9	40
	7–10	30	66	135	54	2400	36	700	3,300	400	10	40
Males	11–14	44	97	158	63	2800	44	1,000	5,000	400	12	45
	15–18	61	134	172	69	3000	54	1,000	5,000	400	15	45
	19–22	67	147	172	69	3000	54	1,000	5,000	400	15	45
	23–50	70	154	172	69	2700	56	1,000	5,000		15	45
	51+	70	154	172	69	2400	56	1,000	5,000		15	45
Females	11–14	44	97	155	62	2400	44	800	4,000	400	12	45
	15–18	54	119	162	65	2100	48	800	4,000	400	12	45
	19–22	58	128	162	65	2100	46	800	4,000	400	12	45
	23–50	58	128	162	65	2000	46	800	4,000		12	45
	51+	58	128	162	65	1800	46	800	4,000		12	45
Pregnant						+300	+30	1,000	5,000	400	15	60
Lactating						+500	+20	1,200	6,000	400	15	80

[a]The allowances are intended to provide for individual variations among most normal persons where they live in the United States under usual environmental stresses. Diets should be based on a variation of common foods in order to provide other nutrients for which human requirements have been less well defined. See text for more detailed discussion of allowances and of nutrients not tabulated here.

[b]Kilojoules (kJ) = 4.2 x kcal.

[c]Retinol equivalents.

[d]Assumed to be all as retinol in milk during the first six months of life. All subsequent intakes are assumed to be half as retinol and half as β-carotene. When calculated from international units as retinol equivalents, three fourths are as retinol and one fourth as β-carotene.

5.7 HOW ARE THE SPECIFIC ENERGY REQUIREMENTS OF THE HOSPITALIZED PATIENT DETERMINED?

The energy administered to a particular patient depends on the individual's disease process and the physician's decision to:

1. Maintain weight or minimize weight loss (therapy utilized in a traumatized or infected individual with normal body composition at the onset of the illness).
2. Achieve positive caloric balance and initiate weight gain (for restoration of body mass in the debilitated individual).

ACHIEVING ADEQUATE NUTRITION IN NORMAL INDIVIDUALS?

Board, National Academy of Sciences—National Research Council (Designed for

Water-soluble vitamins						Minerals					
Folacin[f] (μg)	Niacin[g] (mg)	Riboflavin (B₂) (mg)	Thiamin (B₁) (mg)	Vitamin B₆ (mg)	Vitamin B₁₂ (μg)	Calcium (mg)	Phosphorus (mg)	Iodine (μg)	Iron (mg)	Magnesium (mg)	Zinc (mg)
50	5	0.4	0.3	0.3	0.3	360	240	35	10	60	1
50	8	0.6	0.5	0.4	0.3	540	400	45	15	70	5
100	9	0.8	0.7	0.6	1.0	800	800	60	15	150	10
200	12	1.1	0.9	0.9	1.5	800	800	80	10	200	10
300	16	1.2	1.2	1.2	2.0	800	800	110	10	250	10
400	18	1.5	1.4	1.6	3.0	1200	1200	130	18	350	15
400	20	1.8	1.5	2.0	3.0	1200	1200	150	18	400	15
400	20	1.8	1.5	2.0	3.0	800	800	140	10	350	15
400	18	1.6	1.4	2.0	3.0	800	800	130	10	350	15
400	16	1.5	1.2	2.0	3.0	800	800	110	10	350	15
400	16	1.3	1.2	1.6	3.0	1200	1200	115	18	300	15
400	14	1.4	1.1	2.0	3.0	1200	1200	115	18	300	15
400	14	1.4	1.1	2.0	3.0	800	800	100	18	300	15
400	13	1.2	1.0	2.0	3.0	800	800	100	18	300	15
400	12	1.1	1.0	2.0	3.0	800	800	80	10	300	15
800	+2	+0.3	+0.3	2.5	4.0	1200	1200	125	18[h]	450	20
600	+4	+0.5	+0.3	2.5	4.0	1200	1200	150	18	450	25

[e]Total vitamin E activity, estimated to be 80% as α-tocopherol and 20% as other tocopherols.
[f]The folacin allowances refer to dietary sources as determined by *Lactobacillus casei* assay. Pure forms of folacin may be effective in doses less than one fourth of the recommended dietary allowance.
[g]Although allowances are expressed as niacin, it is recognized that on the average 1 mg of niacin is derived from each 60 mg of dietary tryptophan.
[h]This increased requirement cannot be met by ordinary diets; therefore, the use of supplemental iron is recommended.

Steps for determining caloric intake in patients:

1. Determine the total caloric requirements of the individual based on height and weight or weight alone (see p. 20).
2. To achieve positive caloric balance and initiate weight gain, predict actual daily caloric requirements (see p. 36). Alternately, measure the oxygen consumption of the patient and determine the actual metabolic requirements (see p. 11).
3. For weight maintenance, provide the energy requirements as estimated or measure (+ 25% to cover requirements of daily activities above basal, see p. 36).

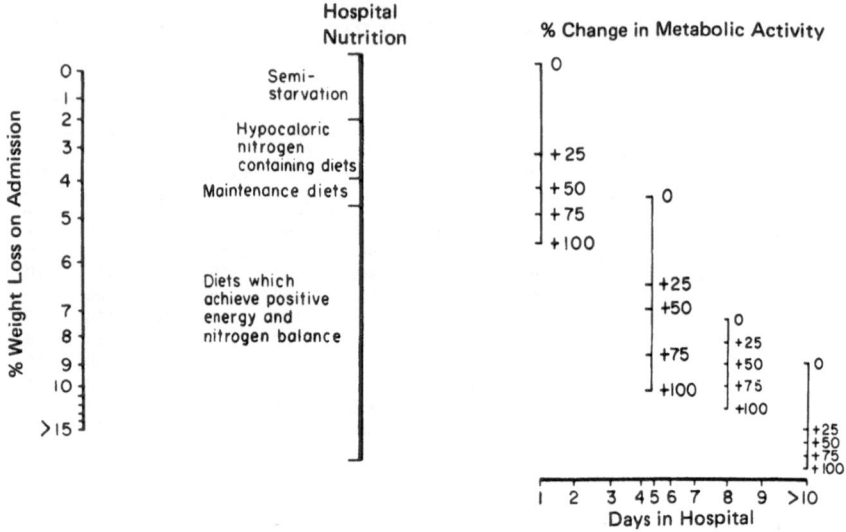

FIGURE 5.1: The type of hospital nutritional intake required by the patient can be determined from this nomogram. Locate the percentage weight loss at the time of admission on the scale at the left (see page 49). Measure or estimate metabolic rate (see page 36, the right-hand scale estimates percent change in basal metabolic activity with various disease processes); locate that point on the scale above the first hospital day. Connecting these points with a straightedge determines the relative energy and nitrogen intake for hospitalized patients on the scale labeled Hospital Nutrition. With time, dietary intake needs to be periodically reassessed and this is done by utilizing the other scales on the right-hand side located above the appropriate hospital day. The physician need not reassess percentage weight loss; use the percentage weight loss that was present on the day of admission. The methods of providing the various types of hospital nutrition are listed below and are discussed in later portions of this chapter.

	Types of feeding		
Route of intake	Semistarvation	Hypocaloric nitrogen-containing diets	Diets which achieve positive energy and nitrogen balance
Oral	Clear liquids	Ad lib diet Hypocaloric tube feedings	Oral diets with supplements High caloric tube feedings Combined enteral-parenteral diets
Intravenous	D-5-W	Amino acid containing hypocaloric diets	Hyperalimentation

4. To achieve weight gain, increase the caloric intake to "safe" levels over and above the estimated or measured metabolic requirements. In most patients, a weight gain of 2 lb/week (positive energy balance of 7000 kcal/week) is a reasonable goal (see p. 43 for prediction of weight gain). Nutritional rehabilitation requires time to restore body mass, and 3–6 weeks of intensive nutritional therapy are often required to replete the depleted patient. Nutritional prophylaxis should be utilized whenever possible, for it is much more efficient to prevent disruption of body mass than be forced to actively replete the wasted catabolic individual.

5.8 HOW SHOULD THE CALORIE REQUIREMENTS BE MET BY SPECIFIC DIETARY PROVISIONS?

Carbohydrate, fat, and alcohol are the primary dietary energy sources. Protein is utilized for building essential functional units of the body and should not serve primarily as a caloric source. The average American diet contains about 45% carbohydrate and 40% fat calories. While the percentage of these two energy-yielding substances may vary from day to day, fat and carbohydrate together supply approximately 85–88% of the daily caloric intake, with the remaining calories provided from protein. This relationship between carbohydrate, fat, and protein in hospital diets is similar to the average daily diet, although increased quantities of protein (up to 20% of the total calories) may be supplied in high-protein diets provided to surgical patients. Carbohydrate in food is provided as oligosaccharides (starch), disaccharides, or monosaccharides (simple sugars), while fat is primarily ingested as triglycerides. Because of its known hepatic toxic effects, alcohol should not be utilized as a primary caloric source.

5.9 WHAT ARE THE ADVANTAGES OF CARBOHYDRATE IN ENTERAL DIETS?

Carbohydrates are essential fuels utilized by glycolytic tissue. Tissues that oxidize fat, like muscle, utilizes carbohydrate when this nutrient is administered as the major dietary fuel. Carbohydrate digestion and absorption are highly efficient in man, and it makes little difference whether the source is cooked starch or simple sugars.

Monosaccharides can be absorbed in high concentrations unless they cause increased motility by their osmotic load. Absorption may be altered in patients with specific enzyme deficiencies (such as lactose intolerance); symptoms produced by the ingestion of a specific sugar can be prevented by eliminating the substance from the diet. Carbohydrate maintains hepatic glycogen stores, which protect hepatocytes during hypoxia or exposure to toxins. Carbohydrate has specific protein-sparing action. Its ease of absorption and nitrogen-retaining effects are the primary factors influencing clinicians to recommend high-carbohydrate—high-protein diets in the care of severely ill patients.

5.10 WHAT ARE THE ADVANTAGES OF INTRAVENOUS DEXTROSE WITH OR WITHOUT INSULIN THERAPY ADMINISTERED TO CRITICALLY ILL PATIENTS?

Over the past 75 years, repeated testimonials have appeared in the literature supporting the use of glucose or glucose and insulin therapy during critical illness. As previously noted, Coleman preferred carbohydrate for its superior nitrogen-sparing capacity. Benn and associates in England, Darrow in this country, and many others administered dextrose and antitoxin in the treatment of diphtheria.[13] Dextrose or dextrose—insulin therapy was also utilized in the treatment of lobar pneumonia and a variety of other infectious processes.

Cardiac function and circulatory status may improve with dextrose administration, an observation made initially by Sodi-Pallares and subsequently confirmed by many investigators in patients with refractory congestive heart failure, hypovolemic shock, or gram-negative septicemia. Liver function may stabilize or improve, but it is not known if this effect is the result of a provision of additional cellular energy or the increased exposure of the hepatocyte to high insulin levels, a hormone thought by some to induce hepatic cell regeneration and replication. In recent years, Allison and co-workers[14] in England have stimulated renewed

[13]Martin, E.: *Dextrose Therapy in Everyday Practice*, New York, Paul B. Hoeber, 1937.
[14]Allison, S. P., Hinton, P., and Chamberlain, M. J.: Intravenous glucose-tolerance, insulin, and free fatty acid levels in burned patients. *Lancet*, 2:1113, 1968.

interest in glucose—insulin administration, reporting the protein-sparing and potassium-retaining effects of this therapy in a wide variety of disease processes. In burn patients with infection, dextrose—insulin infusions resulted in a prompt natriuresis and nonosmotic diuresis. The movement of glucose into the cell is thought to restore the ATP-dependent sodium—potassium pump, which may become energy-deficient during critical illness. Failure of the cell pump results in an increased accumulation of intracellular sodium and water, often referred to as the "sick cell syndrome."

Curreri and associates[15] confirmed the intracellular cation disequilibrium in critically ill patients, and noted that supracaloric feedings administered to extensively injured patients returned the abnormally elevated erythrocyte cation concentration to normal. Further studies confirmed a decrease in active erythrocyte membrane cation transport; restoration of sodium—potassium cell pump activity was achieved by the provision of carbohydrate in the diet. McDougal and associates[16] have extended these studies, demonstrating that hepatic transport of indocyanine green dye (a marker incorporated by active hepatic membrane transport) is improved with the addition of carbohydrate to the parenteral feedings of extensively burned patients.

5.11 WHAT ARE THE HAZARDS OF HIGH-CARBOHYDRATE DIETS? ... OF INTRAVENOUS GLUCOSE?

1. High concentrations of simple sugar in the gastrointestinal tract are an osmotic load, which may cause increased peristalsis and diarrhea.
2. High carbohydrate intake by the enteral, parenteral, or combined routes may cause hyperglycemia, hyperosmolality, and an osmotic diuresis, resulting in dehydration and hypovolemia. Patients with elevated blood-glucose levels as a result of a disease process, obesity, or diabetes are particularly vulnerable to severe

[15]Curreri, P. W., Wilmore, D. W., Mason, A. D., Jr., Newsome, T. W., Asch, M. J., and Pruitt, B. A., Jr.: Intracellular cation alterations following major trauma: Effect of supranormal caloric intake. *J. Trauma, 11*:390, 1971.

[16]McDougal, W. S., Wilmore, D. W., and Pruitt, B. A., Jr.: Glucose dependent hepatic membrane transport in nonbacteremic and bacteremic thermally injured patients. *J. Surg. Res., 22*:697, 1977.

hyperglycemia and the subsequent fluid and electrolyte imbalances when given diets that contain glucose. All patients receiving high-carbohydrate diets, whether by the enteral or parenteral route, should be frequently monitored for hyperglycemia and glucosuria. When present, the intake of carbohydrate should be reduced and/or exogenous insulin administered.

3. Carbohydrate stimulates insulin elaboration which decreases peripheral release of amino acids. Large quantities of dietary carbohydrate without or with inadequate quantities of protein may result in hepatic dysfunction (iatrogenic kwashiorkor). High-carbohydrate feedings should always be accompanied by the intake of adequate dietary protein.

4. Glucose solutions are slightly acid, and the low pH has been implicated as a cause of thrombophlebitis associated with peripheral venous infusion.

5. Glucose and amino acids react in solution (the Maillard reaction). With time or heat, the mixtures become darkened as a result of the glucose—amino-acid complex. Hence, the mixtures have a limited shelf life, cannot be autoclaved, and must be mixed shortly before use. This complexing has been implicated in binding of trace minerals, particularly zinc, which is excreted in increased quantities in the urine.[17]

5.12 WHAT IS THE IDEAL INTRAVENOUS SUGAR? WHAT ARE THE RATES OF UTILIZATION OF VARIOUS SUGARS IN INTRAVENOUS DIETS?

The rate-limiting factor during intravenous delivery of a carbohydrate is determined by the rate in cellular membrane transport. If a sugar is not transported from the blood into the cell and utilized, then, with time, plasma concentrations will exceed the tubular threshold of the kidney, resulting in an osmotic diuresis. The rates of utilization of various carbohydrates and sugar alcohols are shown in Table 5.3. Although it was thought that fructose would provide an insulin-independent sugar for utilization in diabetics or during stress

[17] Freeman, J. B., Stegink, L. D., Meyer, P. D., Fry, L. K., and Denbesten, L.: Excessive urinary zinc losses during parenteral alimentation. *J. Surg. Res., 18*:463, 1975.

Table 5.3   Rates of Utilization for Various Carbohydrates and Sugar Alcohols

Substrate	Infusion rate (g/kg/hr)	Utilization rate (mg/kg/hr)	Calories (kcal/kg/hr)
Glucose	1.5	1.390 ± 30	5.3
Fructose	1.5	1.409 ± 25	5.3
Xylitol	0.5	483 ± 10	1.9
Galactose	0.3	290 ± 10	1.1

Adapted from: Heuckenkamp, P.-U., and Zöllner, N.: The comparative metabolism of carbohydrates administered intravenously. *Nutr. Metab., 14,* Supp. 58, 1972.

states associated with glucose intolerance, this, in fact, is not the case because fructose is converted to glucose by the liver. Fructose also causes several problems: serum phosphorus falls, hepatic ATP decreases, and serum lactic acid rises. Uric acid and bilirubin also increase.

Sorbitol is frequently utilized in other countries, but its osmotic effect on the brain may produce cerebral edema. It is metabolized to fructose, and produces metabolic sequelae similar to fructose administration. Xylitol is a pentose hydroxyalcohol that bypasses insulin-dependent glucose pathways, but alterations in liver function and other side effects have limited its use. Intravenous glucose is the cheapest and most effective carbohydrate for intravenous administration.[18] Others have suggested that carbohydrate combinations be utilized (insulin- and non-insulin-dependent sugar mixtures), but the effect of these "cocktails" is difficult to evaluate.

5.13   WHY IS DIETARY FAT DESIRABLE? ... UNDESIRABLE?

Fat provides the greatest amount of energy per unit weight of any fuel. Slightly less than half of the fat consumed in the diet is derived from butter, margarine, oils, and shortening; about one-third of dietary fat comes from meats, and the remainder from foods such as nuts, cereal, and poultry and dairy products other than butter. Dietary fat adds greatly to the palatability of food, and meals composed of standard foodstuffs are extremely difficult to prepare unless the diet contains about 30% of its calories as fat. Almost

[18]Rowlands, B. J., Giddings, A. E. B., and Clark, R. G.: Carbohydrate infusion in surgical patients: A therapeutic dilemma. *Acta Chir. Scand. Supp., 466*:44, 1976.

two-thirds of all dietary fat comes from animal sources and about a third from vegetable sources. Lipid calories are primarily triglycerides with fatty acids containing chain links of 16 to 18 carbons, and only a small percentage of the fatty acids are polyunsaturated. Dietary lipid maintains our own body fat stores, which serve as endogenous thermal underwear, insulating against cold ambient environments. Fat stabilizes, supports, and protects vital structures, provides fat-soluble substances such as vitamins essential for body metabolism, and contributes to structural components of biological membranes that partition and protect the intracellular or subcellular milieu from the surrounding environment.

The absorption of fat is complex because it is insoluble in water. Triglycerides must be degraded into fatty acids, and monoglycerides combine with bile salts to form soluble micelles, and are then transported into the intestinal epithelial cell, after being separated from the bile salt at the mucous cell membrane. The cell then reforms the triglycerides and assembles them into chylomicrons, which are transported by way of the intestinal lymphatics. The intestinal uptake of fat may be limited by any one of a number of steps and, hence, fat malabsorption may occur with a wide variety of gastrointestinal abnormalities associated with critical illness.

When the proportion of fat and other energy in the diet exceeds the usual energy demands of the body, increased body weight (positive energy balance) results. In our society, overeating is associated with obesity; fats (triglycerides and cholesterol) and their carrier lipoprotein complexes may increase in the blood stream. These serum abnormalities have been associated with an increased incidence of atherosclerosis and myocardial infarction. Dietary modification is often effective in improving the abnormal lipid concentrations in familial, genetic, or dietary-induced disease. Lipid abnormalities are frequently a contraindication for the provision of increased quantities of dietary fats in hospital diets. Infusion of intravenous fat emulsion is similarly contraindicated in patients with abnormalities in fat metabolism.

5.14 WHAT IS ESSENTIAL FATTY ACID DEFICIENCY? HOW IS IT TREATED?

While the major portion of fat stores may arise from *de novo* synthesis, an essential quantity of polyunsaturated fat cannot be synthesized in the body, but is necessary for optimal nutrition. When fat is excluded from the diet, carbohydrate may be readily converted to fatty acids and stored as triglyceride. In 1927, Evans and Burr[19] revealed that exclusion of fat from the diet of rats prevented satisfactory growth and development. Subsequent studies demonstrated that fat-free diets in animals resulted in scaling of the skin, loss of hair, emaciation, impaired reproductive capacity, increased intake of food and water, increased metabolic rate, and early death. These symptoms could be reversed by providing a small amount of fat in the diet, and it was later determined that linoleic acid was the essential fatty acid dietary component.

Hansen and co-workers[20] fed healthy infants five proprietary milk mixtures, adequate in protein, minerals, and vitamins but with varying fat and linoleic acid content. Two diets were found inadequate in linoleic acid, and a high proportion of babies fed these mixtures developed dry, thickened, desquamated skin. The skin lesions rapidly disappeared in the addition of linoleic acid to the formula. In 1971, Collins and his associates[21] described essential fatty acid deficiency in an adult male who had undergone massive intestinal resection and was maintained solely by fat-free intravenous nutrition therapy for 100 days. This patient developed a skin rash in association with biochemical features of polyunsaturated fatty acid deficiency. The signs of the deficiency were reversed with the intravenous administration of a soybean oil emulsion containing linoleic acid. However, the clinical features of the deficiency state, particularly the skin rash, are rarely seen until after several months or more of a fat-deficient diet. Thrombocytopenia, increased hemolysis, and impaired wound healing are associated clinical features which occur with the skin lesions.

The biochemical manifestations of essential fatty acid deficiency are accentuated by increased metabolic demands, associated with growth in children or hypermetabolism following injury or infection in adults. The chemical findings are characterized by abnormally low levels of essential polyunsaturated fats in the

[19]Evans, H. M., and Burr, G. O.: New dietary deficiency with highly purified diets. *Proc. Soc. Exper. Biol. Med., 24*:740, 1927.

[20]Hansen, A. E., Stewart, R. A., Hughes, G., and Soderhjelm, L.: The relation of linoleic acid to infant feeding. *Acta Pediat., 51*(supplement 137), 1962.

[21]Collins, F. D., Sinclair, A. J., Royle, J. P., Coats, D. A., Maynard, A. T., and Leonard, R. F.: Plasma lipids in human linoleic acid deficiency. *Nutr. Metab., 13*:150, 1971.

serum or red cell membrane, associated with a compensatory increase of saturated fatty acids.[22] These alterations may be expressed as an absolute level or a ratio of the triene and tetraenoic fatty acids present. The ratio rises during the deficiency state, and may be used as a guide to follow the response to polyunsaturated fatty acid replacement therapy. In addition, one fatty acid (5,8,11-eicosatrienoic acid) is virtually absent from normal tissue, but appears during essential fatty acid deficiency.

Most hospital diets, tube feedings, and chemically defined or synthetic formulas contain an adequate quantity of polyunsaturated fat for stable, resting man. Deficiency can be prevented by supplying approximately 4% of the caloric requirements as polyunsaturated fat. This quantity of fat can be included in the diet in patients receiving long-term parenteral nutrition by administering an intravenous fat emulsion rich in polyunsaturated fatty acids, such as soybean oil emulsion, or by providing small amounts of polyunsaturated fat (safflower oil) daily by the enteric route.

5.15   WHAT ARE MEDIUM-CHAIN TRIGLYCERIDES? HOW DOES THEIR METABOLISM DIFFER FROM LONG-CHAIN FATTY ACIDS?

Medium-chain triglycerides are one form of neutral lipid which contains fatty acid molecules with a chain length varying from 6 to 12 carbon atoms. While these triglycerides occur in foods as natural lipids, they are most commonly obtained as a manufactured oil (containing principally C:8 and C:10 fatty acids) and serve as a food supplement or additive. Medium-chain triglycerides are more easily and more rapidly hydrolyzed and absorbed than triglycerides of long-chain fatty acids (C:16 and C:18). They are rapidly hyrolyzed in the absence of pancreatic lipase, are digested and absorbed well in the absence of bile salts or in the presence of reduced intestinal absorptive surface area, and are principally absorbed into the portal vein. Because they accompany carbohydrates and amino acids in the portal venous system, their absorption is not dependent upon intramucosal production of chylomicrons. Thus, they are useful food

[22]Holman, R. T.: Essential fatty acid deficiency. *Prog. Chem. Fats Other Lipids,* 9:275, 1968.

additives when there is a defect in the hydrolysis, absorption, or transport of fat.

Medium-chain triglycerides are transported to the liver in the portal venous blood as medium-chain fatty acids, and most of these fatty acids are catabolized in the liver to carbon dioxide, ketones, and acetate.[23] The remainder of the medium-chain fatty acids that are not catabolized are converted to long-chain fatty acids and esterified to triglyceride. Thus, very little medium-chain triglyceride is found in the lipid stores of the body. Medium-chain triglycerides stimulate insulin elaboration, a unique characteristic of these fatty acids, which may be related to carbon chain length or the portal venous transport. Long-chain fatty acids which are packaged in chylomicrons and transported via the lymphatic system do not elicit the same insulinogenic effect.

5.16   WHAT ARE THE SIDE EFFECTS ASSOCIATED WITH ADMINISTRATION OF INTRAVENOUS FAT EMULSIONS? WHAT ARE THE CONTRAINDICATIONS FOR INFUSING FAT EMULSION?

ADVERSE EFFECTS[24]

1. Pyrogenic reaction, which occurs in less than 1% of the infusions.
2. Occasional alterations in coagulation and thrombocytopenia.
3. Hyperlipemia, especially with rates of infusion which exceed 3 g/kg/day or administration of the emulsion to patients with abnormalities in lipid metabolism associated with altered clearance of fat from the blood stream.
4. Impairment in liver function may rarely occur associated with jaundice, elevated SGOT, and BSP retention.
5. Alteration of pulmonary diffusion capacity which will impair oxygen transport across the pulmonary membrane. This is associated with abnormal clearance of fat from the blood stream or rapid administration; this complication may also occur in

[23]Greenberger, N. J., and Skillman, T. G.: Medium-chain triglycerides. *New Eng. J. Med.,* *208*:1045, 1969.
[24]Grotte, G., Jacobson, S., and Wretlind, A.: Lipid emulsions and technique of peripheral administration in parenteral nutrition. *In* Fisher, J. E. (Ed.): *Total Parenteral Nutrition.* Boston, Little Brown, 1976, p. 335.

patients with abnormalities in fat metabolism. Similar studies in injured patients with increased fat clearance do not demonstrate alterations in pulmonary function.

6. Fat overload syndrome associated with some of the early emulsions which caused anorexia, fever, headache, abdominal and back pain, and nausea and vomiting. Impaired liver function, hepatosplenomegaly, and delayed clotting were also observed. This syndrome has not been observed in patients receiving the newer emulsions.

7. Intravenous fat pigment deposits in the liver occur in both animals and man. The brown pigment forms in the Kupffer cells and is associated with microgranulomata formation. Vitamin E administration is thought to reduce the microgranulomata formation.

CONTRAINDICATIONS

1. Abnormalities in lipid transport and metabolism.
2. Diabetes mellitus.
3. Liver disease.
4. Blood coagulant deficiency and thrombocytopenia.
5. Severe pulmonary disease.

5.17   HOW ARE THE NUTRITIONAL EFFECTS OF DIETARY PROTEINS ASSESSED?

A variety of techniques have been employed to assess the effect of nutritional intake on body maintenance and growth. These measurements include nitrogen balance, assessing the body amino acid pools, measurement of growth and weight gain, quantitative and qualitative assessment of tissue proteins, anthropomorphic and/or body compositional measurement of body protein, and quantification of plasma protein concentrations. From the standpoint of daily clinical assessment of patients, there are limitations in all these techniques. Many methods of assessment require sophisticated laboratory support, often relying on biopsy material for analysis.

Serum proteins are maintained in the normal range until marked erosion of body protein occurs.

The easiest and most reliable indication of the effect of protein intake is nitrogen balance. This measurement only reflects total body protein gains and losses and does not indicate the site of synthesis or specific site of organ deposition (muscle, liver, wound). Yet, nitrogen equilibrium or positive balance obtained during adequate balanced nutritional intake is usually associated with appropriate distribution of the stored protein during maintenance or rebuilding of the body cell mass.

5.18   WHAT IS NITROGEN BALANCE? WHAT IS CUMULATIVE NITROGEN BALANCE? WHAT ARE THE ERRORS IN THE MEASUREMENT?

Protein balance is most commonly determined by using nitrogen as the marker to determine balance. Protein is converted to the appropriate quantity of nitrogen by dividing protein in grams by 6.25:

$$\frac{\text{Protein in grams}}{6.25} = \text{Nitrogen in grams}$$

Nitrogen balance is nitrogen intake minus nitrogen loss from the body or:

$$N_{balance} = N_{in} - N_{out}$$

where N_{in} is the dietary nitrogen (determined from food composition tables or by food analysis) and

$$N_{out} = N_{urine} + N_{stool} + N_{skin} + N_{wound} + N_{nasogastric\ and/or\ fistular}$$

Stool nitrogen rarely exceeds 1–2 g/day if diarrhea is not present, and skin losses range between 0.1–0.4 g/m^2/day for most individuals. In the usual individual without abnormal skin or wound losses, skin plus stool nitrogen losses do not exceed 2 g/day. Urea accounts for 80–90% of the urinary nitrogen lost. By adding an additional 20% to urinary urea measurements (urine urea concentration x 24-hr urinary volume), an approximation of urinary nitrogen losses can be made, 2 g added for stool and skin losses, and nitrogen balance approximated:

Nitrogen loss in g/day = Urinary urea nitrogen in mg/100 ml

x urinary volume in liters/day ÷ 100

+ 20% of urinary urea loss +2 g

Although this may be an overestimation of nitrogen loss, especially in patients without stool loss who are receiving intravenous feedings, the nitrogen equilibrium or balance obtained using this technique will be in error in favor of actual protein retention (Fig. 5.2).

The error of nitrogen balance is always in the positive direction, with positive balance favored by food intake which does not occur, loss of urine, and unexplained or underestimated nitrogen losses from the body. Cumulative nitrogen balance is the addition of daily balances over a predetermined time period. Since the error term always favors a positive nitrogen balance, cumulative nitrogen balance cumulates a constant positive error; the calculated data thus appear more favorable for nitrogen retention and protein synthesis.

Finally, protein or amino acids administered may be converted to urea but not excreted. The BUN gradually rises, and unless balance is corrected for urea accumulation (total body water x blood urea nitrogen concentration), the retained urea will again favor positive nitrogen balance.

5.19   HOW IS NITROGEN BALANCE AFFECTED BY NITROGEN INTAKE? ... BY ENERGY INTAKE?

Nitrogen equilibrium cannot be achieved without nitrogen intake. If an individual is maintained on an adequate quantity of nonprotein calories and then receives various amounts of nitrogen in the diet, the relationship between nitrogen intake and nitrogen balance can be established (Fig. 5.3). As nitrogen intake increases, nitrogen balance moves toward equilibrium and then becomes positive.

If the nitrogen loading experiment is repeated while the patient is maintained on a fixed but inadequate quantity of energy to achieve caloric equilibrium, the relationship between energy intake

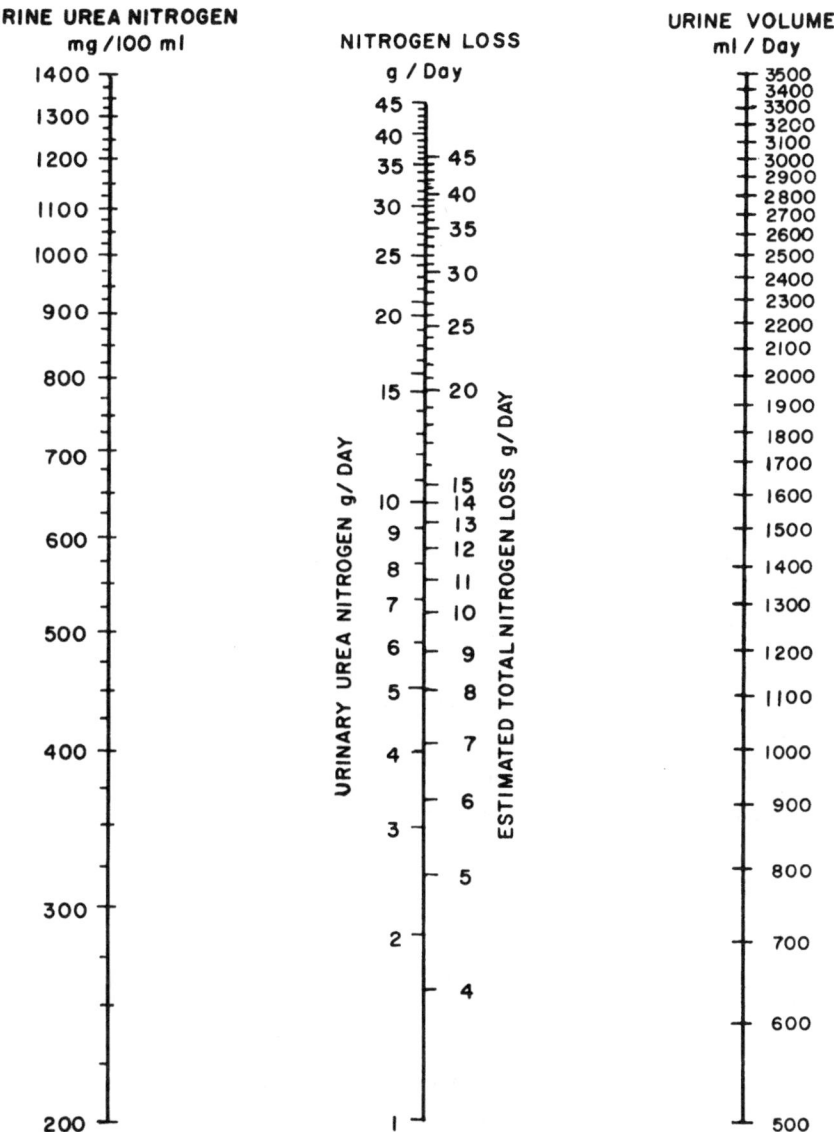

FIGURE 5.2: Nitrogen loss may be estimated from this nomogram. Locate urea nitrogen concentration on the left-hand scale and 24-hr urine output on the right-hand side. By connecting these points with a straightedge, total urea nitrogen or the 24-hr estimated nitrogen loss is determined. Subtracting this value from nitrogen intake yields nitrogen balance.

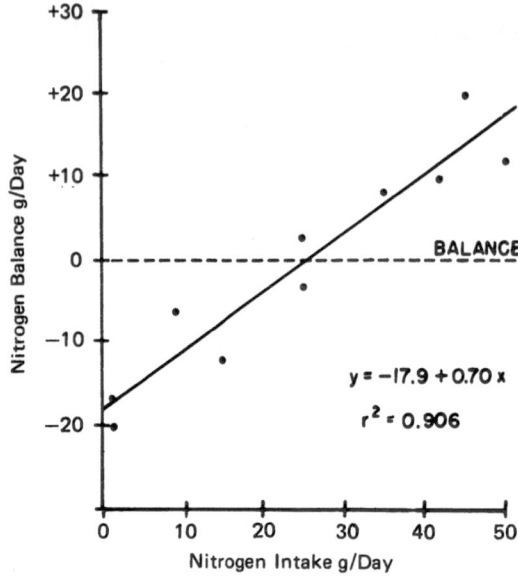

FIGURE 5.3: Varying protein intakes were administered in the random order shown below, while the patient received a constant nonprotein caloric intake which exceeded energy requirements. The effect of nitrogen intake on nitrogen balance is plotted. The point of intersection between the best-fit line and the zero balance line is the nitrogen required to achieve equilibrium. With administration of larger quantities of nitrogen, nitrogen balance will approach an upper limit or plateau.

Estimation of Nitrogen Requirements for Equilibrium in Burned Patients[a]

Day of Study	1	2	3	4	5	6	7	8	9	10
Nitrogen intake (g/day)	1	15	25	45	25	9	35	42	50	1
Nitrogen loss (g/day)	18	27	22	25	28	15	27	32	38	21
Nitrogen balance (g/day)	−17	−12	+3	+20	−3	−6	+8	+10	+12	−20

[a] Adapted from: Soroff, H. S., Pearson, E., and Artz, C. P.: An estimation of the nitrogen requirements for equilibrium in burned patients. *Surg. Gynecol. Obstet.*, *112*:159, 1961.

and nitrogen balance is determined (Fig. 5.4). Increasing the quantity of energy in the diet improves nitrogen balance. On a fixed protein intake, the energy content of the diet is the limiting factor that determines nitrogen balance.[25] The corollary to this rule is that on a fixed energy intake the quantity of nitrogen in the diet becomes the limiting determinant of nitrogen balance.

[25]Calloway, D. H., and Spector, H.: Nitrogen balance as related to caloric and protein intake in active young men. *Amer. J. Clin. Nutr.*, *2*:405, 1954.

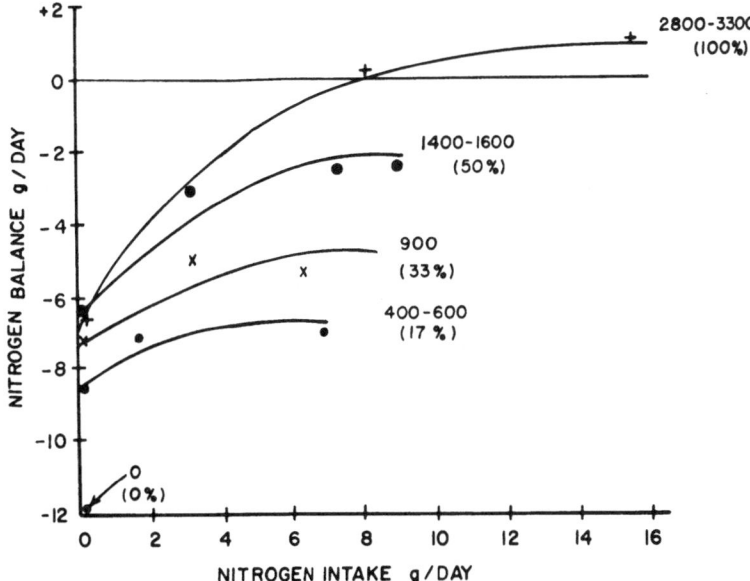

FIGURE 5.4: Nitrogen balance increases with the addition of energy or nitrogen to the diet. The range of calorie intake is listed to the right of each isobar. The number in parentheses below each calorie intake value expresses total calorie intake as a percentage of total daily metabolic expenditure. Data collected by Calloway and Spector: *Amer. J. Clin. Nutr.*, 2:405, 1954.

5.20 WHAT ARE THE LABILE PROTEIN STORES? WHAT IS MEANT BY VISCERAL PROTEIN?

Studies of nitrogen balance in man demonstrate that over a period of several days an individual can adjust his urinary nitrogen excretion to achieve equilibrium over a wide range of nitrogen intakes. When dietary protein is reduced, protein is lost before a new equilibrium is achieved; this protein is thought to arise from organs with high rates of protein turnover or come from free amino acid pools, which are found in intracellular stores in the body. Some sites of deposition of the most labile protein are in the viscera (liver, pancreas, and mucosa of the intestinal tract); other tissues (skeletal muscle) respond less rapidly,[26] while other tissues, such as brain and connective tissue, undergo little change in protein content with starvation. These rapidly fluctuating protein pools have been referred to as "labile

[26]Erik, V., Bergstöm, J., and Fürst, P.: Influence of the postoperative state on the intracellular free amino acids in human muscle tissue. *Ann. Surg.*, 182:665, 1975.

protein stores" (reserve protein) and account for the early nitrogen loss which occurs following starvation or trauma. The labile protein stores are depleted during starvation, and, hence, nitrogen loss is diminished in the depleted patient following injury or operation.

With starvation or injury, amino acids are moved from the carcass (skeletal muscle) to the viscera to support liver function and protein synthesis. Protein-free high-carbohydrate diets blunt this translocation and deprive the liver of essential amino acids. With increased mobilization of fatty acids from adipose tissue, the triglycerides are synthesized in the liver. Amino acids are required to form an apoprotein, which combines with triglyceride in a lipoprotein complex and transports fat from the liver to the periphery. In the absence of amino acids, transport is impaired and fatty liver infiltration occurs. This is frequently observed in kwashiorkor or following long-term administration of glucose-containing protein-free diets.

5.21   HOW ARE AMINO ACIDS METABOLIZED FOLLOWING ORAL FEEDING? ... FOLLOWING INTRAVENOUS FEEDING?

Elwyn studied dogs fed a large meat meal[27]; 57% of the amino acids that entered the liver were converted to urea, 6% formed plasma protein, 23% left the liver as free amino acids, and the remaining 14% presumably remained in the liver for synthesis of liver protein.

In man, plasma concentration of amino acids ranges from 35 to 70 mg/100 ml (alpha amino nitrogen of 4–8 mg/100 ml). Approximately 85% of plasma amino acids leaves the blood stream in 5–15 min. Muscle serves as a large reservoir of amino acids, and these pools are maintained for hours after ingestion of a protein meal. However, free amino acids account for less than 1% of the amino acids in the body. Our total body protein turnover is supported by amino acids in the blood, and it has been estimated that the protein turnover rate in the average man is approximately 300 g/day. Survival time for all protein in the body is about 80 days. In general, extracellular protein has a short half-life: albumin, for example, has a

---

[27]Elwyn, D. H.: The role of the liver in regulation of amino acid and protein metabolism. *In* Munro, H. N. (Ed.): *Mammalian Protein Metabolism*, Vol. 4. New York, Academic Press, 1970, p. 523.

half-life of 10 days, while that of skeletal muscle protein is several months. The labile protein appears to be part of the rapid-turnover protein pool.

It would be thought that the amino acids administered by vein — bypassing the gut and portal circulation — would be handled in a different way. Estimates by Munro suggest that the essential amino acid requirements are quite similar when comparing intravenous administration with enteral feedings.[28] Nonessential nitrogen appears to pass more rapidly into the muscle protein and less readily into liver although further evaluation of this apparent difference is needed. Parenterally administered amino acids are well within the capacity of peripheral uptake, and normal or subnormal levels of plasma amino acids have been observed within a few minutes after terminating an amino acid infusion.

Although intravenous amino acids may be mobilized in a slightly altered manner, there is little doubt that parenterally administered nitrogen-containing substances form the building blocks for protein synthesis. In a series of classic studies by Madden and Whipple,[29] essential amino acids (as described by Rose) were administered by the parenteral route to protein-depleted dogs. Synthesis of new plasma protein occurred. Similar results were obtained with administration of amino acid mixtures by clysis or injection or infusion of the solutions into the peritoneum. Positive nitrogen balance was obtained in dogs and patients with administration of amino acids by the intravenous route, while nonprotein calories were provided by enteral feedings.

Dudrick and associates[30] provided the first demonstration that normal growth and weight gain could be achieved by the administration of all nutrients exclusively by vein. Using paired litter-mate beagle puppies, total calorie and nitrogen requirements were infused continuously by the intravenous route, and the effect was compared with orally fed control animals. Normal growth and

[28]Munro, H. N.: Basic concepts in the use of amino acids and protein hydrolysates for parenteral nutrition. *In: Symposium of Total Parenteral Nutrition*, American Medical Association, 1972, p. 26.

[29]Madden, S. C., and Whipple, G. H.: Amino acids in the production of plasma protein and nitrogen balance. *Amer. J. Med. Sci, 211*:149, 1946.

[30]Dudrick, S. J., Wilmore, D. W., Vars, H. M., and Rhoads, J. E.: Long-term parenteral nutrition with growth, development, and positive nitrogen balance. *Surgery, 64*:134, 1968.

development occurred in animals supported exclusively by vein for 60—210 days, and normal serum protein levels were present in the dogs fed by the parenteral route. Similarly, positive nitrogen balance in adults and growth in babies was achieved by utilizing this technique of total intravenous feedings.

5.22   IS INFUSED PLASMA OR ALBUMIN UTILIZED AS DIETARY PROTEIN?

If parenterally administered plasma protein is retained in the intravascular compartment, it undergoes gradual degradation, and yields nitrogen-containing residues (amino acids and peptides) which are the intermediate or end-products of protein degradation. Early studies in patients and animals demonstrated that positive nitrogen balance can be obtained when infused plasma is the only source of nitrogen intake. However, these studies were criticized because of the belief that transfused plasma proteins are not metabolized rapidly enough to be of value, and that the apparent positive nitrogen balance is spurious and represents an increase in plasma protein pool, rather than utilization for synthesis of lean body mass. These arguments were refuted in 1956, when Allen, Stemmer, and Head reported that normal growth and development were obtained in puppies given 12 g intravenous plasma protein daily as their only source of dietary protein.[31] Paired litter-mates received comparable nonprotein oral calories, with control animals fed 65 g oral protein, 12 g oral protein, and no protein. The puppies maintained for 99 days on intravenous plasma as their only source of protein achieved a gain in height and weight equal to or exceeding that of the litter-mates receiving the same quantity of protein as horsemeat or liver by mouth. Nitrogen balance studies demonstrated positive balance in these animals, and the authors concluded that intravenous plasma appears to be an excellent source of protein for nutrition. In contrast, studies of the nutritive value of transfused red cells demonstrate that this nitrogen source fails as a nutritional protein. While plasma protein should not be administered as a nutritional

[31] Allen, J. G., Stemmer, E., and Head, L. R.: Similar growth rates of litter mate puppies maintained on oral protein with those on the same quantity of protein as daily intravenous plasma for 99 days as the only protein source. *Ann. Surg., 144*:349, 1956.

protein source, it should be appreciated that the intravenous plasma infused to correct hypoproteinemia may in part be utilized for protein biosynthesis and maintenance and repletion of lean body mass.

5.23 HOW IS THE EFFICACY OF VARIOUS PROTEINS ASSESSED? WHAT IS THE BIOLOGIC VALUE OF PROTEIN?

The biologic value of protein is that fraction of absorbed nitrogen retained for body growth and maintenance. In the case of intravenously administered amino acids or hydrolysates, it is the ratio of nitrogen retained to that quantity of nitrogen administered. Proteins containing a low percentage of essential to nonessential amino acids have low biologic value. Similarly, protein with a low concentration of a single amino acid or with a marked imbalance in the ratios of amino acids demonstrated limited efficiency. Because protein of high biologic value is the most efficient and able to provide the optimal balance of essential building-blocks for protein synthesis, high biologic protein should be the major protein source in hospital diets.

Table 5.4   Biological Value of Protein Determined by
Nitrogen Balance

	Growing rat	Mature human
Egg albumin	97	91
Beef muscle	76	67
Casein	69	56
Wheat gluten	40	42

Adapted from: Mitchell, H. H.: *In* Albenese, A. A. (Ed.): *Protein and Amino Acid Nutrition.* New York, Academic Press, 1959, p. 11.

5.24 HOW ARE THE DIETARY REQUIREMENTS FOR PROTEIN DETERMINED? HOW DO THEY RELATE TO CALORIC INTAKE? WHAT IS THE NITROGEN:CALORIE RATIO?

Dietary protein requirements are determined two ways: (1) measure all loss on a protein-free diet, or (2) determine the minimal quantity of nitrogen necessary to achieve nitrogen equilibrium. The first

Table 5.5   Protein Requirements

Subject	Weight (kg)	BSA (m²)	Protein (g/kg/day)	Protein (g/day)	Calories (kcal/day)	Nitrogen: calorie ratio
Infant	9	0.25	2	18	972	1:337
Child	30	1	1.2	36	2400	1:416
Adult	70	1.73	0.8	56	2700	1:301
Adult (postop)	70	1.73	1.5	105	1800	1:107
Adult (stress)	70	1.73	2.25	160	3600	1:140

technique assumes that dietary nitrogen is necessary to replace the losses, but nitrogen equilibrium is not achieved when this quantity of nitrogen is replaced in the diet, and protein requirements are underestimated. The second approach more readily approximates dietary needs, and requirements have been established by this method for children, adults, and traumatized individuals.

The ratio of nitrogen to total energy intake in normals during nitrogen equilibrium is approximately 1:350. Because protein economy decreases with most critical illnesses, the optimal ratio between fed protein and calories is altered. The nitrogen to calorie ratio of 1:150 is thought optimal in seriously ill patients by most investigators, although the ratio may range between 1:100 and 1:200 (Table 5.5).

5.25 HOW DO CARBOHYDRATE AND FAT INFLUENCE NITROGEN BALANCE?

Increased intake of energy usually improves nitrogen retention and nitrogen balance. The effect of fat and carbohydrate varies, and depends on whether (1) the energy source is administered at the same time as the protein or at a different time, (2) fat and carbohydrate are consumed alone or with dietary protein, (3) the additional energy is added to a maintenance diet (classic surfeit or excess feeding) or a hypocaloric feeding, and (4) the metabolic and nutritional state of the individual is abnormal.

In general terms, fat and carbohydrate may be substituted for one another during adequate protein feedings,[32] but there are some exceptions to this general rule. Carbohydrate exerts a more efficient

[32]Munro, H. N.: Carbohydrate and fat as factors in protein utilization and metabolism. *Physiol. Rev., 31*:449, 1951.

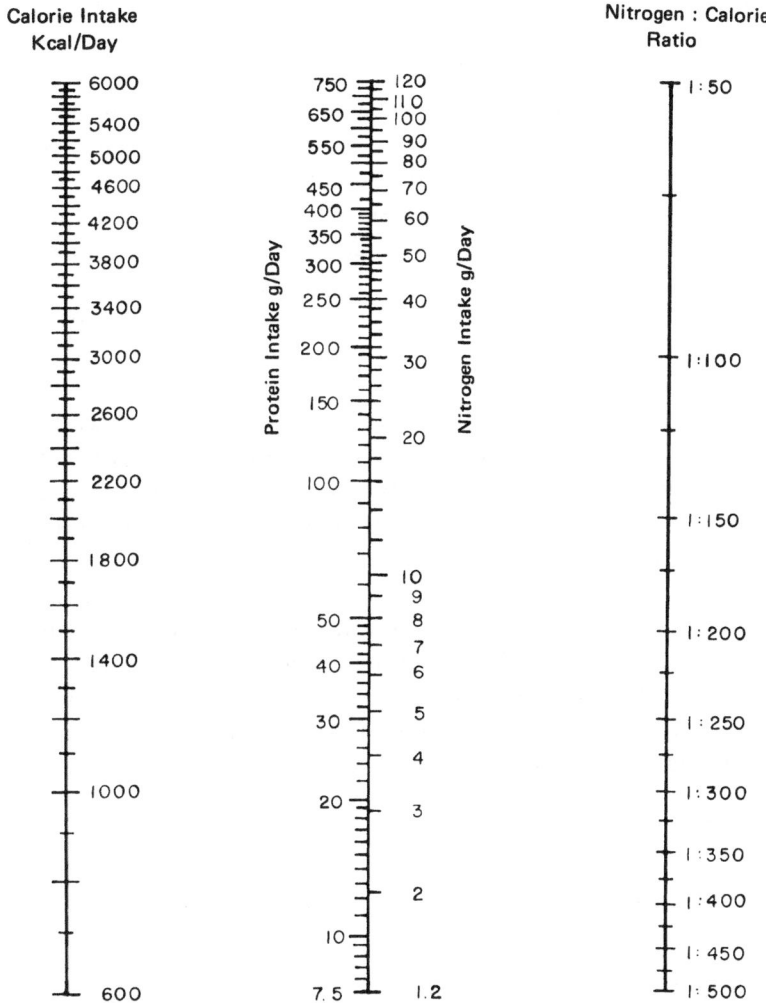

FIGURE 5.5: By relating nitrogen intake to calorie demands, the quantity of protein in the diet is determined. Estimating calorie intake (p. 180), locate this point in the left-hand scale and the nitrogen:calorie ratio on the right-hand scale at 1:150. Connecting these points with a straightedge will determine on the middle scale the quantity of protein required. With patients in simple resting starvation, a higher nitrogen:calorie ratio can be used.

protein-sparing effect when substituted for fat during hypocaloric feedings.[33] Oral or intravenous fat alone does not exert the protein-sparing effect observed with carbohydrate when administered to a subject on a protein-free diet.

The reduced nitrogen excretion observed with infusion of only 10% soybean oil emulsion is minimal and can be accounted for by the free glycerol contained in the emulsion.[34] In hypermetabolic patients infused with a constant dose of amino acids (11.7 g/m^2 of nitrogen per day), a rapid decrease in nitrogen excretion occurred with carbohydrate administration. Comparable doses of fat calories failed to exert a similar effect.[35] As the dose of carbohydrate calories increased, nitrogen excretion decreased. Addition of insulin to the high-carbohydrate infusions further blunted nitrogen loss.

Jeejeebhoy and associates found no alteration in nitrogen excretion after a period of adaptation when intravenous fat was substituted for carbohydrate in starved—adapted patients with chronic gastrointestinal disease (average weight of these patients was 20% below expected norms).[36] The difference in these studies may be reconciled by the fact that hypermetabolic patients have neurohormonal signals which accelerate gluconeogenesis and override the ability of the body to adapt metabolically to starvation by conserving nitrogen and decreasing energy expenditure. In the critically ill patient, intravenous fat is a satisfactory source of essential fatty acids, and provides additional calories to meet energy requirements, thus stabilizing body fat mass and/or increasing body weight; fat should not be administered to the exclusion of carbohydrate in the hypermetabolic critically ill patient. At least two-thirds of the measured or predicted metabolic requirements should be provided by glucose calories in the hypermetabolic critically ill patient.

[33]Munro, H. N.: General aspects of the regulation of protein metabolism by diet and hormones. *In* Munro, H. N., and Allison, J. B. (Eds.): *Mammalian Protein Metabolism*, Vol. 1. New York, Academic Press, 1964, p. 382.

[34]Brennan, M. F., Fitzpatrick, G. F., Cohen, K. H., and Moore, F. D.: Glycerol: Major contributor to the short term protein sparing effect of fat emulsions in normal man. *Ann. Surg., 182*:386, 1975.

[35]Long, J. M., Wilmore, D. W., Mason, A. D., Jr., and Pruitt, B. A., Jr.: Effect of carbohydrate and fat intake on nitrogen excretion during total intravenous feeding. *Ann. Surg., 185*:417, 1977.

[36]Jeejeebhoy, K. N., Anderson, G. H., Nakhooda, A. F., Greenberg, G. R., Sanderson, I., and Marliss, E. B.: Metabolic studies in total parenteral nutrition with lipid in man. Comparison with glucose. *J. Clin. Invest., 57*:125, 1976.

5.26   HOW IS NITROGEN EXCRETION ALTERED WITH CHANGES IN ENERGY EXPENDITURE?

An increase in the excretion of urinary nitrogen occurs in man during heavy work. This may happen because of acceleration in the breakdown of food protein rather than as the result of an increase in endogenous metabolism, as nitrogen excretion is significantly greater when work is performed during the period of absorption as contrasted to the postabsorptive period. Similarly, cold exposure increases nitrogen excretion in animals and man. The elevated metabolic rate associated with disease processes accounts for an increased excretion of urinary nitrogen (Fig. 5.6). Thus, nitrogen balance depends on food intake (quantity of nitrogen in the diet and the quantity of energy in the diet) and the basal metabolic rate of the individual.

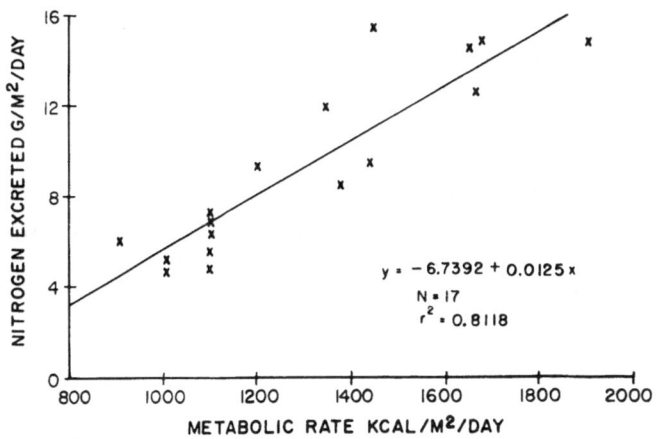

FIGURE 5.6: Nitrogen excretion increases with metabolic activity. Patients received 15 g nitrogen/m^2/day with total calories equaling metabolic rate.

5.27   WHAT ARE THE ESSENTIAL AMINO ACIDS? WHAT IS THE PROPORTION OF ESSENTIAL TO NONESSENTIAL NITROGEN REQUIRED IN A DIET?

The essential amino acids are protein building-blocks which cannot be synthesized by the liver, and hence are essential dietary components (Table 5.6). Nonessential amino acids are synthesized in the liver primarily by transamination, a process that attaches

Table 5.6   Minimum and Recommended Intakes of Essential
Amino Acids for Normal Man When Diet Furnishes Sufficient
Nitrogen for Synthesis of Nonessentials

Amino acid	Minimum daily requirement (g)	Recommended daily intake (g)
L-Tryptophan	0.25	0.5
L-Phenylalanine (tyrosine)	1.10	2.2
L-Lysine	0.80	1.6
L-Threonine	0.50	1.0
L-Valine	0.80	1.6
L-Methionine (cysteine)	1.10	2.2
L-Leucine	1.10	2.2
L-Isoleucine	0.70	1.4

From: Rose, W. C.: Amino acid requirements of man. *Fed. Proc.,* 8:546,
1949.

nitrogen to available carbon skeletons. In addition to the essential
amino acids, extra nitrogen must be provided in the diet to achieve
nitrogen equilibrium, but this may be fed as urea, ammonium
chloride, or a single amino acid. The liver will then convert this extra
nitrogen to nonessential amino acids.

The essential amino acids have been assessed by their impact on
nitrogen balance; addition of a single essential amino acid to a diet
deficient in the component results in a prompt rise in nitrogen
retention that is much greater than the increase which can be
explained by the increase in dietary nitrogen. Although amino acids
have been categorized as essential and nonessential, all amino acids
present in a protein must be available for protein synthesis. Absence
or decreased concentration of a specific amino acid required for
protein synthesis results in that substance limiting synthesis. Hence,
the specific amino acid is referred to as a "limiting" amino acid for
protein synthesis.

The proportion of essential to nonessential nitrogen in the diet
is affected by age and the nutritional state of the individual. Children
require about 40% of the nitrogen as essential amino acids while
adults need only half as much. The "regrowing" adult (regaining
weight) or traumatized individual is thought to have amino acid
requirements similar to those of a growing child.

5.28   HOW DO ESSENTIAL AMINO ACIDS ALONE AFFECT NITROGEN BALANCE IN RENAL FAILURE? IS UREA REUTILIZED FOR PROTEIN SYNTHESIS?

Rose and associates found that as little as $1-2$ gN/day as essential amino acids were necessary for nitrogen equilibrium when other sources of dietary nitrogen and adequate calories were available in the diet. They observed that in rats, ^{15}N urea was incorporated into tissue protein when essential amino acids and calories were provided in the diet.[37] When an additional source of protein was added to the diet, the urea isotope was not recovered from tissue. That the enzymatic hydrolysis of urea by the bacterial flora within the gut participated in the release of nitrogen for protein synthesis was demonstrated by Levenson and co-workers.[38] Approximately $25-40\%$ of ^{14}C urea was incorporated into tissue protein of normal rats, but no incorporation of the tagged urea was observed in germ-free animals. The urea degradation in the gut in humans is about 4 g/day, and the bacterial urease liberates ammonia and carbon dioxide which enter the enterohepatic system and are transported to the liver. The liver transaminates the nitrogen to form nonessential amino acids or it is recycled into the Krebs urea cycle. Nonessential amino acid recycling is dependent on the lack of dietary amino acids and the availability of carbon skeleton (alpha-keto precursors) to accept the nitrogen.

Utilizing these experimental findings, uremic patients were given low-protein diets containing a high percentage of essential amino acids or nonessential amino acids $(1-2$ gN/day) along with adequate calories.[39,40] There was clinical improvement of uremic symptoms, stabilization or a decrease in blood urea concentrations, an increase in lean body mass, and a decrease in total body urea production. The essential amino acid formula (13.1 g of the eight essential amino acids per liter of solution) has been administered intravenously with hypertonic glucose (1400 nonprotein calories per

[37]Rose, W. C., and Dekker, E. E.: Urea as a source of nitrogen for the biosynthesis of amino acids. *J. Biol. Chem.*, 223:107, 1956.

[38]Levenson, S. M., Crowley, L. V., Horowitz, R. E., and Malm, O. J.: The metabolism of carbon-labeled urea in the germ-free rat. *J. Biol. Chem.*, 234:2061, 1959.

[39]Giovannetti, S., and Maggiore, Q.: A low-nitrogen diet with protein of high biological value for severe chronic uremia. *Lancet*, 1:1000, 1964.

[40]Schloerb, P. R.: Essential L-amino acid administration in uremia. *Amer. J. Med. Sci.*, 252:650, 1966.

liter) to postoperative patients in acute renal failure; the rise in serum urea was decreased, lessening the requirement for dialysis; serum potassium, phosphate, and magnesium were stabilized, and renal function appeared to improve at a more rapid rate.[41] The effect of urea recycling in these patients has been questioned; an alternate explanation is that the essential amino acids decrease the rate of urea production and, at the same time, replenish stores of essential amino acids in protein-deficient subjects.

5.29   WHAT ARE THE ALPHA-KETO ANALOGUES OF THE ESSENTIAL AMINO ACIDS? HOW ARE THEY UTILIZED?

Alpha-keto analogues are compounds which appear structurally very similar to the essential amino acids but the nitrogen has been substituted for an alpha-keto group and they are free of nitrogen (alpha-hydroxy analogues have also been used). When included in the diet, these compounds are aminated in the body and converted to the essential amino acid. Since the nitrogen utilized to convert these compounds to essential amino acids arises from endogenous stores, amino acid requirements may be satisfied in part without administering exogenous nitrogen. Hence, the primary value of the alpha-keto analogues is in the treatment of diseases associated with nitrogen retention; they have been used effectively in the treatment of chronic uremia,[42] markedly reducing the frequency of dialysis. Once the analogues are converted to essential amino acids, they exert their effects by diminishing the rate of urea production and replenishing essential amino acid stores.

5.30   HOW IS LIVER FAILURE AFFECTED BY THE INTAKE OF PROTEIN? HOW CAN HEPATIC COMA BE MODIFIED BY SPECIFIC AMINO ACID THERAPY?

Hepatic failure is usually associated with malnutrition. It appears that the tolerance of the cirrhotic patient is greater to parenteral

[41] Abel, R. M., Beck, C. H., Jr., Abbott, W. M., Ryan, J. A., Jr., Barnett, G. O., and Fisher, J. E.: Improved survival from acute renal failure after treatment with intravenous essential L-amino acids and glucose: Results of a prospective double blind study. *New Eng. J. Med., 288:*695, 1973.

[42] Walser, M., Dighe, S., Coulter, A. W., and Crantz, F. R.: The effect of keto-analogues of essential amino acids in severe chronic uremia. *J. Clin. Invest., 52:*678, 1973.

administration of amino acid than similar amounts of protein given orally, but hepatic encephalopathy frequently occurs when protein intakes exceed 40 g/day. Fisher and associates have documented the abnormal amino acid pattern in the serum of patients with hepatic failure and attempted to normalize these concentrations with specially prepared amino acid solutions.[43] The branched-chain amino acids, leucine, isoleucine, and valine, are low in the plasma and the neutral amino acids, phenylalanine, tyrosine, and tryptophan, are normal or elevated. Sepsis, hemorrhage, or operations are stimuli which increase the level of the neutral amino acids (particularly phenylalanine), and an increase in neutral amino acids is observed in other catabolic states. It is suggested that competition occurs between the branched-chain amino acids and the neutral group for penetration of the blood—brain barrier. For example, brain serotonin concentration is determined not only by the plasma concentration of tryptophan but by the ratio of this amino acid to other plasma amino acids: tyrosine, phenylalanine, leucine, isoleucine, and valine.[44] In addition, increased concentrations of phenylalanine may alter transport of precursor amino acids for synthesis of brain dopamine and catecholamines. The level of neurotransmitters in the brain may be determined in part by the abnormal concentrations of plasma amino acids in liver-failure patients.

Attempts to normalize the plasma amino acid pattern in animals and men by infusing a specially prepared amino acid solution with hypertonic glucose have resulted in striking reversal of the symptoms of hepatic coma. Reversal of the coma was noted with infusion of the solution high in branched-chain amino acids and low in concentrations of phenylalanine, tyrosine, and tryptophan; similar effects were not observed with the administration of standard amino acid solutions. Although the results are preliminary, it appears that large quantities of protein (>100 g/day) administered by specialized amino acid solution may now be given to cirrhotic patients in hepatic coma with reversal of the neurological sequelae. These patients can now receive adequate nutritional support.

[43] Fisher, J. E., Rosen, H. M., Ebeid, A. M., James, J. H., Keane, J. M., and Soeters, P. B.: The effect of normalization of plasma amino acids on hepatic encephalopathy in man. *Surgery, 80*:77, 1976.

[44] Fernstrom, J. D., and Wurtman, R. J.: Brain serotonin content: Physiological regulation by plasma neutral amino acids. *Science, 178*:414, 1972.

5.31   WHAT ARE THE VITAMIN REQUIREMENTS IN NORMAL INDIVIDUALS? . . . IN CRITICALLY ILL PATIENTS? HOW ARE THEY BEST PROVIDED?

Vitamins are organic compounds which, in minute quantities, serve as cofactors for essential biochemical reactions.[45] Vitamins are generally classified as fat- (A, D, E, K) or water-soluble compounds (B complex and C). Fat-soluble vitamins are stored in the body in limited amounts, but deficiencies may occur if fat absorption is impaired. Water-soluble vitamins are not stored in appreciable quantities and must be ingested frequently to prevent depletion (Table 5.7).

Vitamins A and D taken in excess may be toxic, but the other vitamins taken in excess of body requirements appear to be quantitatively excreted. Major injury or stress increases the requirements for Vitamin C, niacin, thiamine, and riboflavin. Liver concentrations of Vitamin A also decline but rarely to levels of deficiency. The extent of malnutrition, antibiotic therapy, and administration of antineoplastic agents may influence the tissue levels and metabolism of vitamins. Vitamin requirements are met by a balanced diet; oral supplements may be administered when necessary. If gastrointestinal absorption is inadequate, vitamin requirements should be satisfied by parenteral administration.

5.32   WHAT MINERALS AND TRACE ELEMENTS SHOULD BE PROVIDED IN DIETS FOR THE CRITICALLY ILL PATIENT?

Minerals make up about 5% of the body weight. Their role in basic physiologic processes is unique and essential for the maintenance of cardiac function, mineralization of the skeleton, actions in nerve and muscle, membrane regulation of water balance and metabolism, and participation in energy transformation. The major minerals such as sodium, potassium, calcium, phosphorus, magnesium and their salts of sulfate and chloride comprise approximately three-fourths of the inorganic material in the body; a number of "trace elements" comprise less than 0.01% of body mass. Provision of minerals is essential

---

[45] For more complete discussion of vitamins, the reader should consult the comprehensive chapters in Goodhart, R. S., and Shils, M. E. (Eds.): *Modern Nutrition in Health and Disease*. Philadelphia, Lea & Febiger, 1973.

Table 5.7   Vitamin Requirements in Normal and Critically Ill Individuals

Vitamin	Biochemical action	Signs of deficiency or toxicity	Clinical history, predisposing deficiency	Requirement[a] Normal[b]	Requirement[a] Moderate injury[c]	Requirement[a] Severe injury[c]
A (Retinol)	Maintains epithelial integrity and retinal pigments	Night blindness, xerosis; toxicity usually associated with food faddism, manifested by malaise, dermatitis, peripheral edema and yellow tint to skin	Protein deficiency, fat malabsorption	5000 IU	5000 IU	5000 IU
D	Metabolism of calcium and phosphorus	Rickets, hypocalcemia; toxicity manifested by elevation of serum calcium and phosphorus, soft tissue calcification and renal calculi	Malnutrition, fat malabsorption	400 IU	400 IU	400 IU
E (Tocopherol)	Antioxidant preventing oxidation of polyunsaturated fatty acids	Hemolytic anemia in children, impaired red cell survival in adults	Fat malabsorption	15 IU	—	—
K (Phylloquinone)	Catalyzes prothrombin synthesis in the liver	Decreased prothrombin time	Prolonged antibiotic therapy, bile fistula, obstructive jaundice	0.4 mg	2 mg	20 mg

Continued

Table 5.7 — Continued

Vitamin	Biochemical action	Signs of deficiency or toxicity	Clinical history, predisposing deficiency	Requirement[a]		
				Normal[b]	Moderate injury[c]	Severe injury[c]
C (Ascorbic acid)	Maintains intracellular matrixes of cartilage, and bone, important in collagen synthesis	Poor wound healing, hemorrhage, infection	Malnutrition	45 mg	75 mg	300 mg
Thiamine (B$_1$)	Decarboxylation of alpha keto acids — requirement proportional to carbohydrate in diet	Beriberi, decreased appetite, cardiomyopathy, neurological symptoms	Alcoholism, sepsis, trauma	1.5 mg	2 mg	10 mg
Riboflavin (B$_2$)	Contributes flavoproteins involved in oxidative process	Cheilosis, bleeding gums, seborrheic dermatitis, magenta-colored tongue	Kwashiorkor, severe malnutrition	1.8 mg	2 mg	10 mg
Niacin	Coenzyme in carbohydrate metabolism	Pellagra, dermatitis, dementia, toxicity manifested by flushing and burning sensations	High-corn diets, diets low or lacking in tryptophan	20 mg	20 mg	100 mg
Pyroxidine (B$_6$)	Participates in a variety of enzyme systems associated with amino acid metabolism	Mental depression, dermatitis, increased excretion of tryptophan metabolites	Malnutrition, pyroxidase antagonists (isoniazid used in treatment of tuberculosis)	2 mg	2 mg	40 mg

	Function	Deficiency symptoms				
Pantothenic acid	Converted to coenzyme A which participates in biological acetylation reactions	Decreased antibody production in man, fatigue, nausea	Severe malnutrition	5–10 mg	18 mg	40 mg
Folic acid	DNA synthesis, transfer of one-carbon units	Megaloblastic anemia	Malnutrition, malabsorption, folic acid antagonist	0.4 mg	1.5 mg	2.5 mg
Vitamin B_{12}	Maintains normal folic acid metabolism, myelin synthesis, reducing agent, participates in metabolism of fat, carbohydrate, and protein	Pernicious anemia, neurological symptoms	Malnutrition, malabsorption, ileal resection, HCl and intrinsic factor also necessary for absorption	3 µg	2 µg	4 µg

[a]Deficiency states may require additional vitamin intake to achieve acceptable tissue concentrations.
[b]Normal requirements based on the 1974 Recommended Daily Dietary Allowances of Food for Men 23–50 Years of Age, Nutrition Board, National Academy of Sciences, National Research Council.
[c]From *Therapeutic Nutrition with Special Reference to Military Situations.* National Academy of Sciences, National Research Council, January, 1951.

to the nutritional and physiologic support of critically ill patients (Table 5.8). The adequacy of mineral support of the major substances may be determined by frequent monitoring of serum levels or assay of other biological fluids or tissues. In general, patients with normal body composition will liberate many intracellular minerals during the catabolic phase of the disease process, and the provision of exogenous trace elements is not essential during a period of brief parenteral nutritional support. In contrast, depleted patients require these substances for normal metabolism; deficiencies will be observed in the inorganic substances that are not included in the diet. Minerals are usually adequately provided in most oral diets or prepared feeding formulas, and most deficiency states are observed during total intravenous infusion. However, even addition of these substances to the parenteral diets may not ensure that they are available for utilization by the body for complexing of several minerals in the solution has been demonstrated (p. 186).

Table 5.8   Minerals and Trace Elements Necessary in Diets for the Critically Ill Patient

Sodium chloride	Administration based on usual fluid and electrolyte therapy.
Potassium	Moves into the cell with glucose and amino acids. Is retained in a ratio of 3 mEq for each 1 g N, unless previous intracellular deficiencies existed. Inadequate administration may be rate-limiting to nitrogen balance.
Phosphorus	The tremendous importance of inorganic phosphate for synthesis of high-energy organic bonds demands an adequate supply of this ion. Deficiencies are reported with parenteral diets free of phosphorus; symptoms include weakness, malaise, anorexia, and bone pain, muscle weakness, hyperventilation, and mental depression. Serum concentrations are markedly reduced and red cell ATP and 2,3 DPG levels fall, causing shifts in the oxyhemoglobin dissociation curve. Phosphorus may be administered as a potassium salt (KH_2PO_4), but is present in some hydrolysates and in soybean oil emulsion. Because phosphorus moves into the cell with nitrogen, and this effect is dependent on the quantity of calories, Sheldon and associate suggest the quantity of phosphate necessary is related to the caloric intake; 20 mEq potassium dihydrogen phosphate is necessary per 1000 IV calories.[a]
Magnesium	Deficiencies observed after 3–4 weeks of deprivation in nutritionally intact individuals. Losses increase with diarrhea or

Continued

Table 5.8—continued

	fistula output. Deficiency frequently observed in alcoholic patients. Acute deficiency associated with hypocalcemia and hypokalemia, accompanied by anorexia, nausea, and vomiting.
Zinc	The body contains 1–2 g zinc, which is an essential cofactor in a variety of enzyme systems. Increased catabolism results in the rapid mobilization of zinc from its intracellular stores and excretion. If zinc is omitted from the diet, particularly during repletion in adults or in the growing infant, deficiency will occur, characterized by diarrhea and mental depression, perioral and perinasal dermatitis, and alopecia. Intravenous infusion of 40–80 mg of zinc sulfate per day will reverse the zinc deficiency state.[b]
Iron	The requirements for iron are well known. However, the lack of response of the bone marrow to iron during critical illness and the normal fall in blood levels which occurs during infection suggest that iron should not be administered during the acute phase of most catabolic disease processes, particularly when associated with infection.[c]
Calcium	Large calcium deposits are present in the body, and normal endocrine mechanisms should function to maintain normal serum levels. In addition, patients who remain in bed increase their urinary and fecal calcium losses, and the added effect of calcium infusion in adults must be undertaken with caution. Infusion of phosphate in large doses will lower serum calcium, and it has been suggested that calcium be included in the nutritional mixture when phosphate is given to prevent signs of hypocalcemia. Low-dose phosphate infusion in patients with normal serum calcium levels does not cause a fall in serum calcium. Calcium is essential to the growing infant.
Copper	Deficiency state demonstrated in long-term maintenance parenteral nutrition.
Iodine, manganese, chromium fluoride, cobalt, and other trace elements	Role not identified in parenteral diets.[d]

[a]Sheldon, G. F., and Grzyb, S.: Phosphate depletion and repletion: relation to parenteral nutrition and oxygen transport. *Ann. Surg., 182*:683, 1975.

[b]Kay, R. G., Tasman-Jones, C., Pybus, J., Whiting, R., and Black, H.: A syndrome of acute zinc deficiency during total parenteral alimentation in man. *Ann. Surg., 183*:331, 1976.

[c]Alexander, J. W.: Nutrition and Surgical Infection, in: *Manual of Surgical Nutrition.* American College of Surgeons, Philadelphia, W. B. Saunders, 1975, p. 394.

[d]Shils, M. E.: Minerals in total parenteral nutrition. *In: Symposium on Total Parenteral Nutrition.* American Medical Association, 1972, p. 92.

5.33   WHAT IS THE COMPOSITION OF THE USUAL HOSPITAL DIET? HOW IS IT ALTERED TO SATISFY SPECIFIC NUTRITIONAL REQUIREMENTS?

The usual hospital diet selected by a patient from a food menu is very similar to the diet which most people eat at home. Most hospital diets contain 70—80 g of protein rather than the recommended 50 g based on the recommended daily dietary allowance (p. 180). This diet is based on the requirements for normals, assuming usual physical activity, and should be altered for patients with weight loss and catabolic illness. A high-protein diet increases protein intake to 100—120 g of protein per day, although the quantity of nitrogen may be modified for the disease process involved (increased for the severely catabolic patient and decreased for individuals with nitrogen retention).

Dietary composition can be further altered by the dietitian to satisfy individual patient requirements. Some of the usual diets provided include:

1. Mechanically soft: for those patients who have difficulty chewing.
2. Bland diet: caffeine, spices, and alcohol have been excluded to prevent irritation of the gastrointestinal tract.
3. Residue-restricted or residue-added diets: for patients with inflammatory disease of the intestinal tract.
4. Modification of the carbohydrate and fat content: for patients with abnormalities in lipid metabolism.
5. Lactose-restricted or lactose-free diets: for patients with known lactase intolerance.
6. Low-sodium or low-calorie diets.

5.34   HOW ARE DIETARY SUPPLEMENTS BEST ADMINISTERED? HOW SHOULD THEY BE GIVEN? WHAT SHOULD BE GIVEN?

Studies in critically ill hypermetabolic patients who can eat demonstrate that food intake from meals is slightly less (approximately 15%) than before the injury, although energy requirements may be twice as great.

Anorexia and food boredom is a significant problem. The hospital diet, adjusted for the patient's previous dietary preferences and taste, is supplemented by interval liquid-nutrient feedings. Newer commercially available products are the nutrient bases for the beverage supplement, and the liquid preparations may be modified in a metabolic kitchen if necessary before presented to the patient. A lactose-free formula (Ensure) is ideal for prevention of posttraumatic lactose intolerance or prevention of diarrhea in patients with known lactase deficiency. Modification of this preparation with a calcium caseinate formula or by the addition of dextrins, medium-chain triglyceride oil, egg-white powder, other powdered protein sources, whole fresh eggs, and a variety of flavors increases caloric density, fortifies protein intake, improves palatability, and provides variety. Commercially available dextrins (Polycose) are added to foods or supplements to increase carbohydrate calories without markedly altering intraluminal tonicity or increasing sweetness. Supplements are offered between meals and at night, and are given instead of water. Fruit juices are offered with medication; thus, all liquid intake contains calories.

5.35   WHAT ARE THE INDICATIONS FOR TUBE FEEDINGS? HOW ARE THEY ADMINISTERED? WHAT ARE THE HAZARDS?

Patients who will not or cannot eat but have a functioning gastrointestinal tract are candidates for tube feedings, either by a nasogastric tube or a gastrostomy. Blenderized diets have been utilized in the past, but their consistency requires a large-caliber tube for administration and they may serve as a medium for bacterial growth. However, blenderized diets are cheap and readily available. Commercial diets are available for administration, but may require nitrogen supplementation in specific patients (Table 5.9). They are sterile and available in unit containers.

The diets may be given as a bolus feeding and, with time, 300–500 ml per feeding may be administered every 2–4 hr, although a dilute diet of 100–200 ml should be administered initially. The feeding should be given through a funnel or a barrel of a large syringe and allowed to flow into the stomach by gravity. The feeding tube should then be rinsed with water, for the diet may coagulate and clot, obstructing the tube.

Aspiration of a feeding formula into the lungs is one of the

Table 5.9   Approximate Composition of Commercially Available Liquid and Defined Formula Diets and Food Supplements

	Volume (ml)	Calories (kcal)	Carbohydrate (g)	Fat (g)	Protein or protein equivalent (g, source)	Nitrogen:calorie ratio	Osmolality (mOsm)	Na (mEq)	K (mEq)
Liquid diets									
Complete B	1000	1000	120	40	40	1:156	517	60	37
Ensure	944	1000	137	35	35	1:179	460[d]	30	31
Nutri—1000	944	1000	100	52	32	1:195	400	22	36
Isocal	960	1000	125[b]	42	32	1:192	350	22	32
Defined formula and low-residue diets									
Vivonex	1000	1000	226	0.1	20 (Amino acids)	1:306	500[c]	37	30
Vivonex HN	1000	1000	210	0.4	42 (Amino acids)	1:150	844	34	18
Flexical	1000	1000	154	34	22 (Casein hydrolysate)	1:286	724	15	38
Precision LR[a]	926	1000	226	0.7	22 (Egg albumin)	1:283	600	27	20
Precision HN[a]	1000	1000	207	0.5	42 (Egg albumin)	1:150	580	41	22

Dietary supplements

Meritene powder with 8 oz milk	240	275	31	9	18	1:95	690	11	20
Meritene liquid	240	240	28	8	14	1:107	560[c]	10	10
Sustacal vanilla powder with 8 oz whole milk	240	318	43	8	19	1:106	—	12	21
Sustacal liquid	240	240	33	5	14	1:104	756	10	13
Sustagen powder in water	240	390	66	4	24	1:104	1170	11	20
Nutramigen	240	160	20	6	6	1:167	—	3	4
Carnation Instant Breakfast	240	267	33	8	14	1:116	—	11	18

[a]Similar to defined formula diets but contains egg albumin as protein source.
[b]Lactose free.
[c]Increases with flavoring.
[d]More concentrated formula provided in Ensure.

most serious hazards which may occur. This complication may be minimized by elevating the head of the bed approximately 30° above horizontal for at least 1 hr following each feeding and aspirating the gastric contents to evaluate the residual before each feeding.

Diarrhea may occur with tube feedings. The fat content of the liquid diets is fairly high and only two diets are lactose-free, so altered gastrointestinal function may be the etiology of the intolerance. Additional water is required with the liquid diet because the diets are hypertonic and create solute loads that result in dehydration if free water is not administered. Diluting the formula, administering it slowly and at room temperature, and utilizing small volumes at first and allowing 3—5 days for gastrointestinal adaptation will usually allow resolution of the diarrhea. If intolerance persists, use of a lactose-free formula or a bulk-free, chemically defined diet should be considered.

5.36   WHAT ARE BULK-FREE, CHEMICALLY DEFINED DIETS? WHEN SHOULD THEY BE UTILIZED?

The chemical diets contain carbohydrate in the form of glucose, oligosaccharides, sucrose, dextrins, and starch or multidextrose, which are the main sources of calories. The nitrogen content of the "elemental diets" is an appropriately proportioned mixture of purified L-amino acids or a mixture derived from the acid hydrolysis of casein, with necessary amino acids added to provide a balanced amino acid pattern. In the Precision formulas, egg albumin, which requires digestion, is the nitrogen source. Vitamins and trace minerals are present, and electrolytes may be added as required (note the low sodium concentrations in Flexical). The diets may be low in fat content, but provide essential fatty acids.

Most chemically defined diets are virtually fat-free and bulk-free, requiring minimal digestion, thus bypassing the need for most of the pancreatic and biliary secretions. Because the elemental diets provide predigested nutrients, they are useful in patients with reduced length of small intestine or with malabsorption. Because stool volume is markedly reduced, these diets may be utilized in patients with enterocutaneous fistulas or inflammatory bowel disease. Diarrhea may occur, but when these diets are administered at a slow continuous rate, at starting concentrations of 10—15% and increased up to, but not exceeding, 25% weight/volume (1 kcal/ml in adults), diarrhea is rare.[46]

Most of the bulk-free diets are unpalatable and must be administered through a small feeding tube to ensure adequate intake. Most liquid dietary preparations are designed for nutritional requirements of normal adults and are usually inadequate in nitrogen when administered alone to critically ill patients. A high-nitrogen elemental diet is available for use in hypermetabolic and depleted patients, but the increased concentration of amino acids further augments the disagreeable smell and increases the organic taste, necessitating tube administration of this diet. However, this has not restricted the use of these diets, and most advocates insert small, soft feeding tubes immediately and start low-volume continuous administration of the dilute dietary solutions (usually one-half strength). Both volume and concentration can be increased with time to achieve caloric intakes that exceed energy demands.

The bulk-free diets can be administered through feeding tubes of small diameter. One unique application of the use of elemental diets is the placement of a 16-gauge polyethylene catheter into the jejunum during an operative procedure on the upper or lower gastrointestinal tract.[47] Immediately following operation, dilute nutrient solutions are infused continuously at low rates, and the volume slowly increased over the next several days to provide the fluid, electrolyte, and nutrient requirements by enterostomy feeding, thus obviating the need for intravenous support of postoperative patients beyond the first several days. A study comparing this technique with intravenous nutritional support has not been reported.

5.37 WHEN SHOULD INTRAVENOUS FEEDINGS BE INITIATED?

The general indications for nutritional support have been previously outlined; if adequate nutrients cannot be administered by the

---

[46]Bury, K. D.: Elemental diets. *In* Fisher, J. E. (Ed.): *Total Parenteral Nutrition.* Boston, Little Brown, 1976, p. 395.

[47]Page, C. P., Ryan, J. A., and Haff, R. C.: Continual catheter administration of an elemental diet. *Surg. Gynecol. Obstet., 142:* 184, 1976.

gastrointestinal tract and nutritional support is indicated, then intravenous nutrition should be initiated. Patients with disease-related weight loss (>10%) admitted to the hospital requiring gastrointestinal operations may be candidates for restoration of body mass in an effort to improve survival and minimize postoperative complications. Intravenous nutrition is indicated in patients with postoperative anastomosis dysfunction, intestinal obstruction, pancreatitis, short-gut syndrome, enterocutaneous fistula, inflammatory bowel disease, acute renal failure with ileus or enteritis and hepatic failure. Mortality has been substantially lowered in infants with catastrophic gastrointestinal anomalies requiring one or more major operative procedures and in newborns with intractable diarrhea who receive parenteral nutritional support. Intravenous nutrition has also been utilized in patients who cannot eat (for example, enteritis secondary to radiation or chemotherapy) or those who will not eat enough (preoperative patients or hypermetabolic patients with severe injury). If the indication for nutritional support is present (would the physician feed this patient if his gastrointestinal tract were functioning?) but the requirements cannot be met by enteral feedings, then parenteral nutrition should be initiated.

5.38   WHAT ARE THE BEST RECOMMENDATIONS FOR INTRAVENOUS NUTRIENT ADMINISTRATION? HOW ARE THE REQUIREMENTS BEST PROVIDED?

There are many variations in the fluid, electrolyte, nitrogen, calorie, and mineral requirements in patients; requirements have been estimated for adults and infants (Table 5.10). The requirement should be modified by the impact of the disease process, specific organ system function, and the nutritional status of the patient (see p. 180).

5.39   HOW ARE HYPERTONIC FLUIDS FOR INTRAVENOUS NUTRITION PLANNED?

1. Determine daily fluid requirement.
2. Determine level of caloric intake (p. 182). Is the object of the diet to increase body weight, maintain weight, or allow weight loss? (The use of hypocaloric diets will be considered later.)

Table 5.10   **Estimated Nutrient Requirements for Adults Receiving Intravenously Administered Diets**

Nutrient	Stock solution method (350 ml 50% dextrose *plus* 750 ml 5% protein hydrolysate in 5% dextrose)		Kit method (500 ml 8.5% Freamine II *plus* 500 ml 50% dextrose)	
			Single unit method	
Volume	1100	ml	1000	ml
Calories	1000	kcal	1000	kcal
Dextrose	212	g	250	g
Hydrolysates	37	g		
Amino acids			42.5	g
Nitrogen	5.25	g	6.25	g
Sodium	7	mEq	5	mEq
Potassium	13	mEq		
Phosphate			10	mEq

Additions to each unit of base solution (average adult):

Sodium (chloride and/or acetate, lactate, bicarbonate)	40–50 mEq
Potassium (acetate, lactate, chloride, acid phosphate)	20–40 mEq
Magnesium (sulfate)	8–10 mEq
Phosphate (potassium acid salt)	12–18 mMol

Additions to only one unit daily:

Vitamin A	5000–10,000	U.S.P. units
Vitamin D	500–1000	U.S.P. units
Vitamin E	2.5–5.0	IU
Vitamin C	250–500	mg
Thiamine	25–50	mg
Riboflavin	5–10	mg
Pyridoxine	7.5–15	mg
Niacin	50–100	mg
Pantothenic acid	12.5–25	mg
Calcium (gluconate)	4.8–9.6	mEq

Optional additions to daily nutrient regimen:

Vitamin K	5–10	mg	
Vitamin B_{12}	10–30	µg	Alternatively may be given IM in
Folic acid	0.5–1.0	mg	appropriate daily or weekly dosages
Iron	2.0–3.0	mg	

Micronutrients such as cobalt, copper, iodine, manganese, and zinc are present as contaminants in hydrolysate solutions, but may be given in plasma transfusion (10 ml/kg) once or twice weekly if desired.

Adapted from: Duke, J. H., Jr., and Dudrick, S. J.: Parenteral feeding. *In: Manual of Surgical Nutrition.* American College of Surgeons, Philadelphia, W. B. Saunders, 1975, p. 297.

3. Fix the nitrogen intake to caloric intake at the appropriate level (1:150). This step is generally programmed by the use of kits for intravenous diet composition.
4. Start by administering 1 or 2 liters of the nutrient solution at a constant continuous rate over the 24-hr period, gradually increasing the volume of nutritional solution infused to maximum levels of fluid tolerance. This should provide an adequate level of calorie intake.

5.40   WHAT PRECAUTIONS SHOULD BE TAKEN WHEN STARTING HYPERTONIC GLUCOSE AND AMINO ACID INFUSIONS?

The hypertonic nutrient solutions are infused by a central venous catheter directed into the superior vena cava. The catheter is placed via the subclavicular or external or internal jugular vein under aseptic techniques that have been well described. The most efficient approach is subclavicular vein puncture. X-ray confirmation of the catheter placement is mandatory before initiation of the nutrient solution infusion.

The initial insulin response of the pancreas may be inadequate if the entire calculated glucose load is infused on the first day. This will result in hyperglycemia and glucosuria. Infusing only 1 or 2 liters of nutrient solution the first several days allows the beta cells of the pancreas to adjust gradually to the increasing glucose load. The physician can observe the patient's response to the initial glucose load and adjust therapy accordingly. With time, increased endogenous insulin elaboration occurs and the glucose load may be further increased; exogenous insulin, if administered, may no longer be necessary.

Finally, a rigid catheter-care protocol must be followed. Catheter-related infection should not exceed 6% with proper catheter care.

5.41   WHEN IS COMPLETE INTRAVENOUS NUTRITION ADMINISTERED BY PERIPHERAL VEIN INDICATED? WHAT ARE THE ADVANTAGES AND DISADVANTAGES OF COMPLETE NUTRITION BY PERIPHERAL VEIN?

With the availability of a 10% soybean oil emulsion for clinical use, complete intravenous nutrition may be administered by peripheral vein. There are limitations to this approach, and they include cost, tonicity of nutrients infused into a peripheral vein, and volume of solution tolerated by the patient. Three diets which can be utilized for intravenous use are shown in Table 5.11.

In 3 liters of solution, these diets will provide maintenance levels of energy in patients in resting starvation. The solutions, if totally mixed, would provide weight/volume concentrations of 8–10%, and tonicity would be increased slightly with the addition of electrolytes, vitamins, and trace elements. Phlebitis and thrombosis frequently are associated with infusion of more hypertonic solution by peripheral vein. The second diet exceeds 60% of the caloric intake as fat, which is the upper limit for the recommended quantity of fat in the diet. Note that the quantity of amino acids is adequate for nitrogen balance in a patient in resting starvation, but provides inadequate protein intake for hypermetabolic patients.

With these formulas, caloric intake can be increased by: (1) increasing volume of infusion; or (2) increasing the concentration of glucose, which would require central venous administration because of the increased tonicity.

Thus, with the present day intravenous formulas in the United States, *maintenance* nutrition may be provided by peripheral vein in patients in resting starvation who do not present contraindications to increased dietary intake of lipid (see p. 191). Weight gain is minimal and nitrogen balance will vary from negative to slightly positive, depending on the catabolic state of the patient (see p. 202). If the patient can eat, peripheral venous nutrition is useful in combined enteral–parenteral feedings in critically ill patients.

5.42   HOW ARE FAT EMULSIONS ADMINISTERED?

The glucose and amino acid solutions are combined in the manufacturing pharmacy with the appropriate minerals and vitamins, divided into equal volume, and placed in two separate units. Each unit containing the glucose–amino acid mix is infused over a 12-hr period. At the same time, the fat emulsion is administered by "piggyback" through a Y connector so that the two solutions mix in the short length of administration tubing proximal to the intravenous needle. By infusing the fat only 20 hr/day (8:00 A.M. to 4:00 A.M.),

Table 5.11   Example of Three Intravenous Diets for Peripheral Vein Administration

Volume	Nutrient solution	Calories	Nitrogen:calorie ratio	Percentage solution	Percentage nutrients in diet		
					Protein	Fat	Carbohydrate[a]
1 liter	10% glucose	400					
1 liter	8.5% amino acids	340					
1 liter	10% soybean emulsion	1100					
3 liters		1840	1:135	7.8	18	55	27
0.5 liter	20% glucose	400					
1 liter	8.5% amino acids	340					
1.5 liters	10% soybean emulsion	1650					
3 liters		2390	1:176	8.7	14	63	23
0.25 liter	50% glucose	500					
1.25 liter	8.5% amino acids	425					
1.5 liters	10% soybean emulsion	1650					
3 liters		2575	1:151	10	16	58	26

[a]Includes glucose solution plus free glycerol added to fat emulsion.

time is allowed for lipid clearance from the blood stream so that an infusion lipemia will not interfere with the diagnostic blood tests drawn in the early morning.

5.43 CAN INTRAVENOUS FAT EMULSION BE UTILIZED AS A COMPONENT IN NUTRITION ADMINISTERED BY CENTRAL VENOUS ROUTE?

Yes, a variety of dietary combinations may be utilized, and some investigators prefer administering 50% of the nonnitrogen calories as fat and the other 50% as carbohydrate. The importance of these combinations is to maintain the nitrogen:calorie ratio at approximately 1:150 and to follow the guidelines previously established for fat emulsion infusion (metabolic rate elevation <25% and no other contraindications to fat infusion [p. 191]). The precautions of proper catheter placement and maintenance still are required. The cost of central venous fat infusion may be the major consideration, preventing extensive use of fat emulsion. A table to aid construction of fat-containing hypertonic diets is given (Table 5.12).

Table 5.12   Fat and Glucose: Guide for Construction of Intravenous Diets

		No fat		1 liter fat		1.5 liters fat	
Total calories	Volume of 8.5% amino acid solution	Volume of 50% glucose	Total volume infused	Volume of 50% glucose	Total volume infused	Volume of 50% glucose	Total volume infused
1500	750	750	1500	100	1850	—	—
2000	1000	1000	2000	300	2300	0	2500
2500	1250	1250	2500	500	2750	200	2950
3000	1500	1500	3000	700	3200	400	3400
3500	1750	1750	3500	900	3650	600	3850
4000	2000	2000	4000	1100	4100	800	4300

5.44 WHAT IS THE EFFECT OF INFUSING HYPOCALORIC SOLUTIONS CONTAINING AMINO ACID ON NITROGEN BALANCE?

Those factors that affect nitrogen excretion include metabolic rate of the patient and calorie and nitrogen intake. Since nitrogen balance is the difference between nitrogen intake and nitrogen loss, and there is always some loss of nitrogen from the body, nitrogen equilibrium and positive nitrogen balance cannot be achieved unless nitrogen is present in the diet. Blackburn[48] has proposed administration of amino acids alone to reduce postoperative negative nitrogen balance, but has contended that this response would occur only if dextrose was omitted from the intravenous diets. Insulin levels fell on the glucose-free diet, promoting fat mobilization and ketosis. Greenberg and associates demonstrated that the protein-sparing effects of the amino acids were a function of the amino acid intake alone and not a result of starvation adaptation.[49] Nitrogen balance did not vary when either glucose or a fat emulsion was added to the parenteral amino acids nor was nitrogen excretion dependent on serum insulin or ketone levels. The impact of hypocaloric carbohydrate addition to intravenous amino acids was demonstrated by McDougal and associates in severely catabolic injured patients.[50] Increasing the nitrogen intake of hypocaloric diets improved nitrogen balance and adding carbohydrate to the amino acid infusion further improved nitrogen balance. Similar studies have demonstrated a dose-related response to larger doses of carbohydrate in normal man and injured patients.

Hypocaloric infusates of amino acid and dextrose are slightly hypertonic and may be infused by peripheral vein. These diets minimize nitrogen loss (rarely, if ever, is positive balance achieved). Because energy intake is inadequate to achieve energy balance, weight loss occurs. Hypocaloric diets are ideal for short-term administration or supplementation of enteral or tube feedings. They should be utilized instead of 5% dextrose solutions if the patient requires more than 4—5 days of IV support, has a normal nutritional status, and is only mildly hypercatabolic. If the physician can predict from the clinical course that balanced nutrition will be required, then the total energy and nitrogen requirements should be administered.

[48]Blackburn, G. L., Flatt, J. P., Clowes, G. H. A., Jr., O'Donnell, T. F., and Hensel, T. E.: Protein sparing therapy during periods of starvation with sepsis or trauma. *Ann. Surg., 177*:588, 1973.

[49]Greenberg, G. R., Marliss, E. B., Anderson, G. H., Langer, B., Spence, W., Tovee, B., and Jeejeebhoy, K. N.: Protein-sparing therapy in postoperative patients. Effect of added hypocaloric glucose or lipid. *New Eng. J. Med., 294*:1411, 1976.

[50]McDougal, W. S., and Wilmore, D. W.: The effect of isotonic intravenous solutions on nitrogen balance. *Surg. Gynecol. Obstet.*, In press.

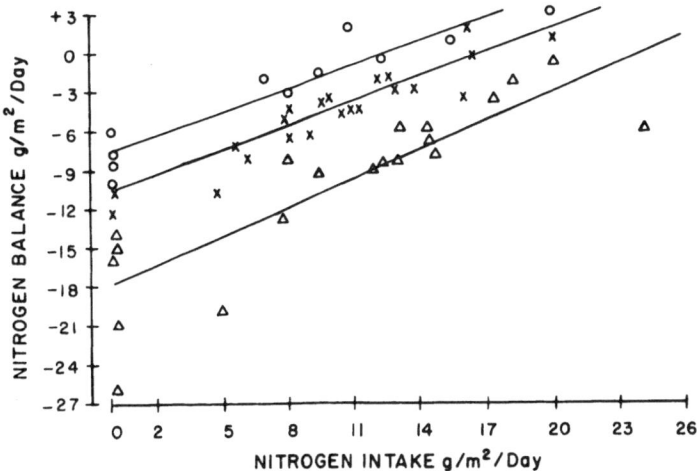

FIGURE 5.7: Increasing nitrogen intake improves nitrogen balance in severely injured patients. Adding glucose to the diet improves nitrogen retention at any level of nitrogen intake. The impact of 60 g of amino acids on nitrogen balance is similar to the impact of administering 60 g of glucose. ○ 120 g glucose/m², x 60 g glucose/m², △ 0 g glucose/m².

5.45   HOW SHOULD A FEBRILE EPISODE DURING CENTRAL VENOUS PARENTERAL FEEDINGS BE HANDLED?

1. Take history and examine the patient. Evaluate all other possible sources of infection.
2. If the findings indicate a non-catheter-related source for the infection (lungs, urinary tract, or wound), continue the infusion and initiate appropriate treatment.
3. If the catheter is suspected as a source of infection, change the infusate and infusion tubing promptly.
4. Culture the infusate, peripheral blood, and blood drawn through the catheter for bacterial and fungal growth.
5. If fever persists 4–12 hr, the catheter should be removed and the tip cultured for bacteria and fungi; the catheter should also be removed if multiple positive blood cultures not related to an obvious source are obtained.
6. A new peripheral intravenous infusion should be started and 5 or 10% glucose administered to avoid hypoglycemia.
7. Appropriate antimicrobial and/or antifungal therapy should be started, based on clinical condition and culture results.

8. Reculture the blood stream after the catheter has been removed and determine the precise cause of sepsis (break in technique, etc.) in order to avoid a similar error in the future.

   If in doubt, remove the catheter.

5.46   WHAT ARE THE METABOLIC COMPLICATIONS THAT OCCUR WITH INTRAVENOUS FEEDINGS? WHAT MONITORING METHODS ARE NECESSARY TO ASSURE SAFE INTRAVENOUS NUTRITION?

A variety of excesses or deficiencies have been associated with total parenteral nutrition. Hyperglycemia, with attendant osmotic diuresis and secondary changes in water and electrolyte metabolism, is always a threat. Conversely, symptomatic hypoglycemia may occur with sudden cessation of the glucose load. Disorders in electrolyte, mineral, and vitamin metabolism may occur if too much or too little of the substances is administered. Proper monitoring is the best method for preventing these complications (Table 5.13).

Other metabolic complications include hyperchloremia, metabolic acidosis (due to excess chloride load), azotemia, hyperammonemia, and essential fatty acid deficiency. Moderate changes in hepatic enzymes may occur but appear transient and often improve despite continuation of the nutritional infusions.

5.47   WHEN SHOULD COMBINED ENTERAL–PARENTERAL FEEDINGS BE ADMINISTERED? HOW?

Parenteral nutrition, as a technique for supplementing oral feedings, is also indicated in the debilitated, malnourished, or thin patient who has limited body fuel stores and inadequate food intake by the enteral route. Even in the face of tremendous energy requirements in the critically ill patient, combined enteral–parenteral feeding techniques can provide more than enough calories and nitrogen to prevent negative energy and nitrogen balance from occurring following injury. The use of the gastrointestinal tract can be assured by utilizing liquid tube feedings administered round-the-clock, using individualized feeding formulas. Parenteral feedings can be modified to contain the volume of fluid and concentration of nutrient to supplement the enteral diet. Parenteral nutrients may be admin-

Table 5.13   Variables to Be Monitored during Intravenous
Alimentation with Suggested Frequency of Monitoring

Variables to be monitored	Suggested frequency	
	First week	Later
I. *Energy Balance:*		
Weight	Daily	Daily
II. *Metabolic Variables:*		
1. Blood measurements:		
Plasma electrolytes		
(Na^+, K^+, Cl^-)	Daily	3 x weekly
Blood urea nitrogen	3 x weekly	2 x weekly
Plasma osmolarity[a]	Daily	3 x weekly
Plasma total calcium and		
inorganic phosphorus	3 x weekly	2 x weekly
Blood glucose	Daily	3 x weekly
Plasma transaminases	3 x weekly	2 x weekly
Plasma total protein and		
fractions	2 x weekly	Weekly
Blood acid–base status	Daily	3 x weekly
Hemoglobin	Weekly	Weekly
Ammonia	2 x weekly	Weekly
Magnesium	2 x weekly	Weekly
2. Urine measurements:		
Glucose	4–6 x daily	2 x daily
Specific gravity or osmolarity	2–4 x daily	Daily
3. General measurements:		
Volume of infusate	Daily	Daily
Oral intake (if any)	Daily	Daily
Urinary output	Daily	Daily
III. *Prevention and Detection of Infection*		
1. Clinical observations (activity,		
temperature, symptoms)	Daily	Daily
2. WBC count and differential	As indicated	As indicated
3. Cultures	As indicated	As indicated

[a]May be predicted from 2 x Na concentration (mEq/liter) + blood glucose
(mg/100 ml) divided by 18.

istered by peripheral or central venous routes. Vitamins and trace
elements are administered by the gastrointestinal tract in patients
who are receiving concomitant enteral feedings. If enteral feedings
are impossible, all essential nutrients should be provided in the
parenteral diet, and frequent blood and urine monitoring performed
to determine precise electrolyte and mineral needs.

5.48   WHAT ADJUNCTIVE MEASURES SHOULD BE INITIATED WITH DIETARY THERAPY?

1. *Administration of Anabolic Hormones.* Human growth hormone, the most potent anabolic agent known, has the unique physiologic role of promoting growth and improving storage of nitrogen, potassium, and phosphorus, and facilitating the transport of amino acids. Administration of growth hormone to nine patients with large thermal injuries, in addition to calories and nitrogen required to meet or exceed predicted energy requirements, resulted in marked augmentation of nitrogen retention, which appeared to be a dose-related response. BUN decreased, blood glucose increased slightly, but more important, serum basal insulin approximately doubled. A close relationship existed between nitrogen balance and basal insulin secretion, and increased insulin augmentation appeared to be the controlling mechanism for the improved nitrogen retention.

2. *Maintenance of an Active Muscle Mass.* Deposition and incorporation of amino acids into skeletal protein is facilitated by muscular activity. Critically ill patients have marked limitations on their activity and require a planned exercise program to maintain an active and functional skeletal mass. With the help of physical therapists, simple isometric exercises can be accomplished while the patient remains in bed or has his extremities immobilized, and these exercises may aid the vitality of the muscles and help restore nitrogen balance across the skeletal muscle bed once caloric and nitrogen equilibrium have been achieved. Technological advances, such as air-fluidized and water beds, provide improved methods for patient care, yet discourage active use of muscle groups. These devices provide the patient with unique suspension systems that simulate the antigravity state, and may increase the breakdown of lean body mass if regular and special exercises are not instituted.

3. *Resolution of the Initiator of the Hypermetabolic Process.* Every effort should be made to resolve the infective process, diminish wound contamination, and/or aid wound healing. Judicious use of antibiotics, operative drainage of abscesses, and well-planned surgical procedures remain the mainstays in limiting postinfective and/or posttraumatic catabolism. Cold ambient temperature,

pain, anxiety, and hypovolemia are potent afferent stimuli that accentuate the metabolic response to injury and infection; these factors can be minimized by careful clinical management. Following resolution of the initiator of the hypermetabolic response, the patient's appetite seems to improve, his spirits rise, and increased exercise is possible. Convalescence heralds a rebuilding of body mass, a gain in weight, and the patient's return to an active and productive life.

Appendix:

Metabolic Support Plan – Using the Metabolic and Nutritional Worksheet

---

Frequent assessment of the patient is necessary to evaluate the success of your nutritional therapy. Use this support plan to determine initial nutritional management, then recalculate the impact of this therapy every 3–5 days in patients with critical illness. Adjustments in dietary support may be necessary to achieve the appropriate and desired results.

Step 1. Enter descriptive characteristics of the patient on the Metabolic and Nutritional Worksheet. (see page 239)

Step 2. Determine body surface area from present weight and height using Fig. 1.6 (p. 21), and enter this figure in blank (2).

Step 3. Find the basal metabolic rate based on the age and sex of the patient in Table 1.7 (p. 22), and enter this value in blank (3).

Step 4. Use Fig. 1.7 (p. 23) to determine the daily basal metabolic rate from body surface area (2) and basal metabolic rate (3).

Step 5. To determine the effect of the disease process on basal metabolic rate, use Fig. 1.11 (p. 36). First estimate the percentage change in metabolic activity associated with a disease process using the right hand scale and enter this value in blank (5a). Then, using daily basal metabolic rate (4), determine the estimated metabolic rate from the nomogram; if metabolic rate is measured, enter this value in blank (5b).

Step 6. Determine the percentage weight loss from Fig. 1.14 (p. 49). If initial weight is unknown, use Table 1.13 (pp. 45–47) for average weights of adults as the initial weight. If body weight has increased because of fluid loading, use 0 percentage weight loss.

Is weight loss limited (0–10%), significant (10–20%), or serious (>20%)? Check the appropriate box.

Step 7. Determine the relative level of calorie intake required for your patient using percentage change in metabolic activity (5a), percentage weight loss (6), and Fig. 5.1 (p. 182). Check the appropriate blank under type of hospital nutrition (7).

Step 8. Now determine the daily calorie requirements for your feeding program. Some guidelines are listed below:

Hypocaloric, nitrogen-containing diets: Provide 400–1800 calories/day, usually 1000–2000 calories below the estimated metabolic rate (5b).

Maintenance diets: These diets achieve energy balance which can be predicted from the estimated metabolic rate plus an additional 25% to account for the energy expended in the hospital during sitting, exercise, and treatment. For this absolute level of calorie intake, read from Fig. 1.11 (p. 36), left-hand side of middle scale.

Positive energy and nitrogen balance: These diets provide calories in excess of the estimated metabolic rate. By adding 1000 calories each day to the estimated metabolic rate, a weight gain of approximately 1.5–2 pounds should be achieved each week.

Step 9. Determine the nitrogen requirements based on a nitrogen:calorie ratio of 1:150 and the daily calorie requirement (8). Use Fig. 5.5 (p. 203), and enter the nitrogen intake in the appropriate blank. Lower nitrogen:calorie ratios may be used in hypocaloric feedings.

Step 10. Choose the type of feeding suitable for your patient and the clinical situation from the following table. Enter the type of feeding in the appropriate space.

Now refer to the appropriate tables for selection of the exact nutrients to be used [Table 5.9 (pp. 218–219) for tube feedings and supplements, Tables 5.11 (p. 226) and 5.12 (p. 227) for parenteral diets]. Enter the nutrient(s) used in the appropriate space (10).

Route	Hypocaloric, Nitrogen-containing	Maintenance or Positive Energy and Nitrogen Balance
Enteral feeding	1. *Ad-lib* food intake from hospital trays 2. Low-volume or dilute tube feedings	1. High-calorie, high-protein diet with between-meal supplements 2. Adequate tube feedings 3. Chemically defined diets
Parenteral feeding	1. Amino-acid-containing peripheral vein infusions	1. Hypertonic glucose and amino acids infused by central venous catheter 2. Fat-containing peripheral venous infusions in non-stressed patients

Step 11. Vitamins, minerals, and essential fatty acids are usually provided in most hospital diets and commercially available tube feedings. These substances may need to be supplemented in infected or severely injured patients fed by the enteral route and should be added to all parenteral diets [see Table 5.10 (p. 223)]. Intravenous fat emulsion (one unit every 2 or 3 days) should be administered as part of the parenteral feeding to all depleted individuals and patients receiving IV fat-free parenteral diets for more than 2–3 weeks.

Step 12. Frequent assessment of the patient is necessary to evaluate the success of your nutritional therapy. Enter the mean daily calorie intake and the weight gain or loss over the past week in the appropriate blanks (you may need to consult your dietitian for the mean daily calorie and nitrogen intake). To assess the impact of the dietary calories on body weight, compare the predicted weight change [see Fig. 1.13 (p. 43)] with the real weight change over a week. If actual weight gain is greater than the predicted weight gain, why? Is it fluid retention? An underestimation of calorie intake? A decrease in metabolic rate? If the patient has lost weight, reassess the percentage weight loss (see *Step 6*). Is weight loss approaching the 10% limit? Should calorie intake be increased? Are you achieving your nutritional goals with this patient?

Step 13. Enter the nitrogen data in the appropriate blanks. Calculate nitrogen balance from the 24-hr urine urea nitrogen and nitrogen intake using Fig. 5.2 (p. 195). To improve nitrogen balance, increase calorie and nitrogen intake and/or employ ancillary measures such as hormonal therapy, increasing ambient temperature, and exercising the patient.

CASE 1.   PERITONITIS IN A PATIENT WITH INFLAMMATORY BOWEL DISEASE

A 40-year-old male is admitted to the hospital with a past history of inflammatory bowel disease, fever, mild abdominal tenderness, and an enterocutaneous fistula. He is 5′9″ tall and weighs 125 pounds. He has eaten poorly for the past month. His usual normal weight was 165 pounds. How much would you feed him now? How?

Follow the instructions on pp. 235–238. The numbered steps correspond to the numbers on the worksheet. First, fill out the facts known about the patient (*Step 1*). In Fig. 1.6 (p. 21), you can use either feet or centimeters, pounds or kilograms. Now calculate total body surface area. Locate 5′9″ on the left-hand scale and 125 pounds on the right-hand scale and connect the two points. It crosses the middle scale at 1.7 m^2. Enter this figure on the worksheet (2). Move to *Step 3*. Locate metabolic rate in Table 1.7 (p. 22). Enter this figure (36.3 kcal/m^2/hr) on the worksheet and move to *Step 4*. Figure 1.7 (p. 23) multiplies the basal metabolic rate (3 on worksheet; locate this value on the left-hand scale of the nomogram) by the surface area (2, right-hand scale) to determine the daily basal metabolic rate (1450 calories/day; enter this number in blank 4).

Determine the impact of the disease [Fig. 1.11 (p. 36)]. This patient has fever, a fistula, and abdominal tenderness, all signs of peritonitis. I estimate his metabolic rate at 20% above basal (enter this figure in 5a), which places the estimated metabolic rate of this patient at 1700 kcal/day (5b).

Determine the percentage weight loss from Fig. 1.14 (p. 49). Move to the *Step 7* nomogram to predict the relative level of energy intake. Connect the percentage weight loss (24% in this patient, so use > 15%) on the left-hand scale of the nomogram [Fig. 5.1 (p. 182)] with the percentage in metabolic activity (20%; locate on the scale

METABOLIC AND NUTRITIONAL WORK SHEET

(1)   NAME_____ AGE_____ SEX_____ DATE_____

     HOSPITAL DAY_____TIME ELAPSED SINCE FOOD INTAKE MAINTAINED BODY WEIGHT_____ DAYS

     PRESENT WEIGHT_____HEIGHT_____WEIGHT BEFORE ONSET OF DISEASE_____

(2)   BODY SURFACE AREA_____m^2

---

(3)   BASAL METABOLIC RATE_____$kcal/m^2/hr$ (5a) % CHANGE IN METABOLIC ACTIVITY_____

(4)   DAILY BASAL METABOLIC RATE_____kcal/day   (5b) ESTIMATED METABOLIC RATE_____kcal/day

---

(6)   % WEIGHT LOSS_____LIMITED_____SIGNIFICANT_____SERIOUS_____
(7)   HOSPITAL NUTRITION   (8) DAILY CALORIE REQUIREMENTS
_____SEMISTARVATION (CLEAR LIQUIDS OR D-5-W)   USE NO LONGER THAN FOUR DAYS
_____HYPOCALORIC, NITROGEN-CONTAINING DIETS
     (ESTIMATED METABOLIC RATE-1000-2000 CALORIES)   _____ kcal/day ⌉
_____MAINTENANCE DIETS (ESTIMATED METABOLIC RATE + 25%)   _____ kcal/day ⌉
_____POSITIVE ENERGY AND NITROGEN BALANCE (ESTIMATED
     METABOLIC RATE + APPROXIMATELY 1000 kcal)   _____ kcal/day ⌋
(9)   NITROGEN INTAKE (BASED ON NITROGEN:CALORIE RATIO
     OF 1:150)   _____ g/day ⌋
     NITROGEN INTAKE FOR HYPOCALORIC DIETS (BASED
     ON 1:75-150 RATIO)   _____ g/day ⌋

(10)

ROUTE	TYPE OF FEEDING	NUTRIENT USED
ENTERAL FEEDING		
PARENTERAL FEEDING		
ENTERAL-PARENTERAL FEEDING		

(11)

	PRESENT IN DIET	NEEDS SUPPLEMENTATION
VITAMINS.	_____	_____
MINERALS	_____	_____
ESSENTIAL FATTY ACIDS	_____	_____

⟶ CHECK ⌋

(12) MEAN DAILY CALORIC INTAKE OVER PAST WEEK   _____ kcal/day

     WEIGHT CHANGE OVER PAST WEEK   _____ pounds

(13) MEAN DAILY NITROGEN INTAKE   _____ g/day ⌉

     URINARY UREA NITROGEN CONCENTRATION _____ mg/100 ml
                                                                                            SUBTRACT
     24-HOUR URINARY VOLUME   _____ ml

     ESTIMATED TOTAL NITROGEN LOSS   _____ g/day ⌋

                                   NITROGEN BALANCE   _____ g/day

Fig. A1. Metabolic and nutritional worksheet.

over the first day in hospital) to determine the hospital diet. In this case, the diet should achieve positive energy and nitrogen balance. The daily calorie requirement (*Step 8*) is:

$$1700 + 1000 = 2700 \text{ kcal} - \text{let's say } 3000 \text{ kcal/day}$$

We would give 20 g nitrogen to achieve a ratio of 1:150 (*Step 9*). In selecting the diet for a depleted patient with a small intestinal fistula, I would start with a central venous parenteral feeding containing hypertonic glucose and amino acids with vitamins and minerals added (*Steps 10* and *11*). Fat should be administered intermittently (one 500-ml unit of fat emulsion every 2 or 3 days will provide the essential fatty acid requirement).

After 1 week of 3000 kcal/day intake, the patient has gained 2.5 pounds. Is this water? No, this is real tissue [see Fig. 1.13 (p. 43), which predicts the amount of weight gain from the energy balance equation).

Urine urea nitrogen is 500 mg/100 ml, and total volume is 2000 ml/24 hr. Estimate nitrogen balance. Following *Step 13*, nitrogen loss is estimated at 14 g/day; the patient is in positive balance of +6 g/day ($20_{in} - 14_{out}$).

CASE 2.   MULTIPLE TRAUMA IN A YOUNG, HEALTHY MALE

A 25-year-old, 195-pound, 6'3" college football halfback is admitted to the hospital following an automobile accident in which he sustained intraabdominal injuries, cerebral contusion, and a femoral fracture. Postoperatively, the patient is on a ventilator. What is your initial nutritional therapy?

Now you solve this problem and see whether we agree:

(2)	Body surface area:	2.2 m^2
(3)	Basal metabolic rate:	$37.5 \text{ kcal/m}^2/\text{hr}$
(4)	Daily basal metabolic rate:	1950 kcal/day
(5a)	Percentage change in metabolic activity:	65%
(5b)	Estimated metabolic rate:	3200 kcal/day
(6)	Weight loss:	0, limited

  (7) Hospital nutrition: Hypocaloric, nitrogen-
                                 containing diets
  (8) Daily calorie requirement: 1200–2200 kcal/day
  (9) Using a ratio of 1:100 would give approximately 15 g
       amino acid nitrogen if renal function is normal.
(10) Parenteral feeding: Amino-acid-containing
                                 peripheral vein infusion.
       I would mix 400 ml 8.5% amino acid solution with 600 ml
       10% dextrose and infuse 3–4 liters/day as indicated by
       fluid requirements.
(11) Supplement needed?   Vitamins, yes—but will not
                                 require all the minerals
                                 necessary for anabolism
                                 (Ca, Mg, Zn, etc.) at this
                                 time.
(12) He gains 2 pounds over the first week. Is this water? (yes).
Reevaluate diet therapy at 5 days postinjury; assume that the
metabolic rate is unchanged:
  (7) Hospital nutrition: Maintenance diet
  (8) Daily calorie requirement: 4000 kcal/day
  (9) Nitrogen intake: 26 g nitrogen
(10) Parenteral feedings   Hypertonic glucose and
                                 amino acids by central
                                 venous infusion.
                                 Approximately two thirds
                                 of the calories should be
                                 carbohydrate; the remain-
                                 ing calories can be fat (see
                                 Step 10).

CASE 3.   A SMALL BURN INJURY IN A DEPLETED WOMAN

A 55-year-old female is transferred to your service on the third
hospital day with a 20% total body surface burn on her lower
extremities. Height is 5'3". She weighs 95 pounds. Her normal
weight was 120 pounds, but has slowly fallen over the past four
months since her husband died.

ANSWERS FOR THE METABOLIC AND NUTRITIONAL WORK SHEET

(2) 1.4 m^2

(3) $33.3 \text{ kcal/m}^2/\text{hr}$

(4)   1100 kcal/day

(5a) 50%

(5b) 1650 kcal/day

(6)   21%, significant

(7)   Positive energy and nitrogen balance

(8)   2700 kcal/day

(9)   18 g

(10) Enteral feeding, high-calorie, high-protein hospital diet with between-meal supplements. Select your supplement from Table 5.9 (pp. 218–219).

(11) Supplement vitamins; the other nutrients are present in the diet.

After 1 week of dietary therapy, the average calorie intake is 3000 kcal/day and the patient has gained 2.5 pounds. Is this water?

(12) No

Her urine contains 725 mg urea/100 ml, and she voids 1700 ml/24 hr. Her nitrogen intake is 24 g/day. Is she in positive balance?

(13) Yes (output 17 g; input $24 - 17 = +7$ g/day; even with increased losses from her wound, which may account for an additional loss of 4 g of nitrogen/day, this patient is still in positive nitrogen balance).

CASE 4.   INTRAABDOMINAL POSTOPERATIVE COMPLICATIONS: EDEMATOUS PATIENT REFERRED TO YOUR SERVICE AFTER 2 WEEKS OF SEMISTARVATION

A 35-year-old male with chronic duodenal ulcer disease underwent vagotomy and pyloroplasty 2 weeks ago. On the fifth postoperative day, he developed a spiking temperature, right upper quadrant pain, and mild hypotension. Abdominal exploration revealed a leak from the duodenostomy, and the pyloroplasty was resutured and drained. The patient continued his febrile course, and three positive blood stream cultures for gram-negative organisms were reported over the following week. The day before referral to your service, his right upper quadrant sump drain output was 1.2 liters/24 hr. Gastrographin instilled through his nasogastric tube revealed a controlled duodenal fistula with no distal intestinal obstruction. No other intraabdominal collection was suspected.

Previous history revealed that this 5'8" man weighed 73 kg before operation. He has received D-5-W throughout his 2 weeks of prior hospitalization. His present weight is 73 kg, although pedal and sacral edema are now present. His serum albumin concentration is 2.1 g/100 ml. His last positive blood culture was 4 days ago, and his highest daily temperature is now 103.5° F.

ANSWERS FOR THE METABOLIC AND NUTRITIONAL WORKSHEET

(2) 1.86 m^2
(3) $36.5 \text{ kcal/m}^2/\text{day}$
(4)   1600 kcal/day
(5a)   40%, based on the fact that this patient has had severe infection
(5b)   2200 kcal/day
(6)   0% — but this weight represents the accumulation of edema fluid.

By estimating his daily calorie intake (3 liters D-5-W/day = 600 kcal/day) and his metabolic rate (5b), his loss of body tissue, independent of fluid, can be approximated [see Fig. 1.13 (p. 43)]. This estimate suggests that the patient is losing at least 1.5 kg/week, or 3 kg since his operation 2 weeks ago. This approximation would suggest that this weight loss is approaching at least 5% [using Fig. 1.14 (p. 49) and a present weight of 70 kg]. Although still limited, this patient's body mass must be vigorously maintained. Resolution of his infection or increasing the calorie intake, or both, will allow positive energy and nitrogen balance to be achieved.

(7)   Positive energy and nitrogen balance
(8)   3200 kcal/day
(9)   21 g/day
(10)   Parenteral feeding — hypertonic glucose infused by central venous catheter: This diet can be administered as 3 liters of the hypertonic solution (500 ml 8.5% amino acids plus 500 ml 50% glucose) with additional fluid requirements provided by peripheral vein infusion of isotonic glucose and electrolyte solutions. Alternately, a liter of fat emulsion can be added to the nutritional infusion to increase the calorie and fluid intake.

(11) Vitamins, minerals, and fat should be supplemented. In addition, albumin, 50 g/day, should be administered to correct the hypoalbuminemia.

CASE 5. PARENTERAL NUTRITION FOLLOWING INJURY AND RENAL FAILURE

A 54-year-old female sustained soft tissue injury and fractures of two long bones and the pelvis from an automobile accident. Despite rapid fluid resuscitation, the patient passed only 10–20 ml of urine each hour. Urologic and roentgenologic examinations demonstrated an uninjured urinary tract, and the diagnosis of acute renal failure was made. After 4 days of intravenous support with D-5-W, her paralytic ileus persisted. She is 5′ tall, weighed 110 pounds before injury, but gained weight to 120 pounds following fluid resuscitation. Her nasogastric tube losses averaged 1 liter/day, and she voided 200–300 ml urine/day. How should she be managed?

ANSWERS FOR THE METABOLIC AND NUTRITIONAL WORKSHEET

(2) 1.50 m^2
(3) $33.3 \text{ kcal/m}^2/\text{day}$
(4)   1200 kcal/day
(5a)   40%
(5b) 1680 kcal/day
(6)   0%, limited
(7)   Maintenance diet
(8)   2080 kcal/day
(9)   Although this patient would require 14 g nitrogen/day if renal function were normal, acute renal failure requires modification of the "standard" nutritional formula. Thus, the renal failure patient requires calories to minimize protein catabolism and the minimal requirement of essential amino acid (or protein of high biological value, — such as egg protein) to aid protein synthesis and/or further limit tissue breakdown. This quantity of protein should range from 2 to 4 g/day (but can be increased as renal function improves or with frequent hemodialysis), and can be provided in intravenous diets

by a commercially available preparation of the essential amino acids. As a second choice, a very dilute solution of the usually used 8.5% crystalline amino acid solution containing both essential and non-essential amino acids may be administered.

(10)   Parenteral feeding — hypertonic glucose and essential amino acids infused by central venous catheter: The volume of fluid administered should be minimized in this edematous patient with minimal urine output. By combining 800 ml 50% glucose with 100–200 ml essential amino acid solution, and infusing 1 liter of this combination per day, more than enough calories can be provided and fluid intake is minimized (most patients will also receive some additional fluid with parenteral medications). Volume may be increased as urine output improves. However, in the diuretic phase of renal failure, more dilute nutritional solutions may be necessary to provide adequate fluid intake and maintain fluid balance. Sodium intake must be adjusted to balance losses; potassium and phosphorus additions may be necessary, but in low concentrations; glucose intolerance should be avoided (by the administration of insulin, either by subcutaneous injections or, more practically, by the addition of insulin to the parenteral nutritional solution), and strict attention to sources of possible sepsis (attention to all portals of entry) is a necessity.

(11)   Supplementation of vitamins and minerals — but with caution. The reader is referred to the recommended requirements for parenteral nutrients in renal failure fluid by Abel.[1]

(12, 13) Although appropriate estimations of alterations in body weight may be made on occasion, the large fluid shifts in these patients often mask body compositional changes. Because of nitrogen retention, possible endogenous urea utilization, and marked fluctuations of the blood urea nitrogen (with and without dialysis), nitrogen balance cannot be determined by *Step 13*.

---

[1] Abel, R. M.: Parenteral nutrition in the treatment of renal failure. *In* Fisher, J. E. (Ed.): *Total Parenteral Nutrition*, Little, Brown, 1976, p. 143.

CASE 6. HEPATIC DYSFUNCTION IN A PATIENT WITH AN ENTEROCUTANEOUS FISTULA RECEIVING INTRAVENOUS FEEDINGS

This 33-year-old female with achalasia underwent surgical repair 3 weeks ago but developed an esophageal fistula. During a second surgical procedure, a left subphrenic abscess was drained and a gastrostomy placed. Although her weight has been maintained for the past 2 weeks with hypertonic glucose and amino acid feedings by central venous catheter, liver function tests are abnormal: alkaline phosphatase, total bilirubin, and hepatic enzymes have all gradually increased. Bile is present in her gastrostomy tube drainage, and tests for hepatitis are negative. Attempts to feed by the gastrostomy tube have been unsuccessful. She is now jaundiced but is afebrile and "feels well."

She is 5'10" and presently weighs 130 pounds. How should she be managed?

ANSWERS FOR THE METABOLIC AND NUTRITIONAL WORKSHEET

(2) 1.74 m^2

(3) $35.0 \text{ kcal/m}^2/\text{hr}$

(4)   1450 kcal/day

(5a)   5% — she is an afebrile postoperative patient without signs of peritonitis or systemic sepsis.

(5b) 1500 kcal/day

(6)   16%, limited, although her initial weight is unknown, predicted weight is 154 pounds.

(7)   Positive energy and nitrogen balance

(8)   2500 kcal/day

(9)   17 g/day

(10)   This patient has progressive hepatic dysfunction associated with a disease process or parenteral nutrition or both. The etiology is unknown, but the liver function abnormalities may be related to (1) an imbalance in carbohydrate load relative to the dose of amino acids administered or (2) two operations, intraabdominal sepsis, and/or associated hepatic perfusion abnormalities (all of which are now presumably resolved). In this

nonstressed patient who requires vigorous nutritional support, we can shift the proportion of nonprotein calories from a predominantly carbohydrate source to a mixed fat–carbohydrate energy source. (In patients without this degree of weight loss, some have proposed "cyclic hyperalimentation" — hypertonic glucose and amino acids administered for 15 hr, then amino acid alone infused over the next 9 hr.[2]) The proposed fat-containing diet can be administered by either the peripheral or central venous route.

In addition, I would favor attempting to feed this patient by the gastrointestinal tract, although gastrostomy feedings were not tolerated. With a well-sealed gastrostomy, a small, weighted catheter could be directed through the gastrostomy and into the duodenum, then gradually advanced into the jejunum. The tube can be started under direct visualization using a pediatric endoscope, inserted through the gastrostomy, or could be manipulated during fluoroscopic visualization. Following satisfactory tube-positioning in the jejunum, a defined-formula diet is started (dilute strength, small volume used initially, then volume and concentration gradually increased), which would provide high portal concentration of nutrients and allow more normal nutrient delivery to the liver. As the enteral feedings are increased, the parenteral feedings could gradually be decreased, but the overall proportion between the fat and carbohydrate energy should be maintained along with a relatively constant daily nitrogen load. The defined-formula diets are also high-carbohydrate diets, so as enteral feedings are increased, carbohydrate is gradually decreased in the parenteral infusion: fat serves as the primary energy source administered by the intravenous route, and this parenteral diet can be administered by peripheral vein.

[2] Maini, B., Blackburn, G. L., Bristrian, B. R., Flatt, J. P., Page, J. G., Bothe, A., Benotti, P., and Rienhoff, H. Y.: Cyclic hyperalimentation: An optimal technique for preservation of visceral protein, *J. Surg. Res.* 20:515, 1976.

CASE 7.   BACTEREMIA IN A PATIENT WITH SEVERE PERITONITIS: MANAGING NUTRITIONAL REQUIREMENTS, HYPERGLYCEMIA, THE INTRAVENOUS CATHETER, AND FEVER

A 39-year-old malpractice lawyer, actively campaigning for mayor, is admitted following his collapse during a political rally. He is hypotensive with signs of peritonitis. Laparotomy reveals a perforated gastric and duodenal ulcer and extensive peritoneal contamination. The perforations are oversewn and his upper abdomen drained. He is maintained on a respirator, has evidence of hepatic and renal dysfunction, and requires large volumes of intravenous fluids, colloid and blood, to maintain adequate organ perfusion. On the seventh hospital day, parenteral feedings are started through a central venous catheter inserted for this purpose. Three days later, the patient develops a spiking temperature to 105°F, urine output increases, urine sugars test 4+, and the blood glucose is reported as 350 mg/100 ml. You are called to "treat the catheter sepsis." What should you do? How should this patient be managed?

The central venous catheter has been in place for only 72 hr, and there are no obvious breaks in maintaining asepsis at the catheter entrance site or in the fluid manufacture. The patient still has signs of peritonitis, and no infection can be traced to the respiratory or urinary tract or the wound (see p. 229 for the steps in managing catheter sepsis). I would discontinue the IV fluids, but not remove the catheter, and replace the parenteral nutritional solution with isotonic glucose, continuing fluids to maintain and restore volume or electrolyte composition and osmolality. Culture the infusate and blood.

The patient's temperature falls in the next 2 hr, and roentgenologic studies suggest a right subphrenic abscess, which is drained posteriorly under local anesthesia. Following drainage, the patient's temperature ranges between 101 and 103°F and the blood glucose is 120 mg/100 ml.

Should the central catheter be removed? This again is a clinical decision. If blood and abscess cultures demonstrate the same organism, and the parenteral fluid demonstrates no growth, then the etiology of the sepsis has been identified. However, if you are unsure about the catheter as a source of sepsis or feel the catheter could be seeded during the bacteremia, then remove it. I would favor removal of the catheter at this time. Parenteral nutrients can be administered for several days by peripheral vein, and the patient's clinical course and blood culture reports will indicate when the blood stream is cleared of infection. When the bacteremia is controlled, a new central catheter can be reinserted and central feedings started.

With reinitiation of the central venous parenteral feeding, the blood glucose rises and glucosuria is present. To control the hyperglycemia, small doses of insulin can be administered subcutaneously, or, alternately, crystalline insulin can be added to the parenteral infusions. Insulin should be administered with caution to prevent episodes of hypoglycemia, which are often undiagnosed in critically ill patients, especially those requiring respiratory support (see p. 92 for discussion of insulin half-life).

Finally, throughout this febrile episode, the patient should be allowed to regulate his body temperature around the new setpoint as long as it is maintained within the 101—103°F range. Aspirin and cooling blankets are not indicated in patients with this level of fever (see p. 73).

CASE 8. EDEMA, HYPOPROTEINEMIA, AND MALNUTRITION FOLLOWING BLUNT ABDOMINAL TRAUMA AND SMALL BOWEL RESECTION

A 42-year-old, slightly obese laborer sustained blunt abdominal trauma in an industrial accident and required abdominal exploration and a 60% distal small bowel resection. He was referred to your service after 12 days of parenteral D-5-W with marked edema, hypoproteinemia (albumin of 1.8 mg/100 ml), and weight loss. Previous attempts to feed by the oral route resulted in severe diarrhea. The patient is 5'10" and now weighs 190 pounds. He is afebrile and convalescing from his operation.

ANSWERS FOR THE METABOLIC AND NUTRITIONAL WORKSHEET

(2) 2.06 m^2
(3) $36.3 \text{ kcal/m}^2/\text{day}$
(4)   1800 kcal/day

(5a) 0; this patient is convalescing in the postoperative state.

(5b) 1800 kcal/day

(6)   0, limited; although this patient must have lost body mass over the past 2 weeks, this is masked by fluid retention.

(7)   Maintenance diet; although this patient is slightly obese, it is better to stabilize his body weight, conserve protein stores, attempt to unload the retained fluid, and provide adequate enteral nutrition before a controlled reduction program is attempted.

(8)   2250 kcal/day

(9)   16 g/day

(10) Our strategy will be to maintain the patient on parenteral feedings while the optimal enteral diet is determined. He will then be weaned off parenteral feedings and maintained on his oral diet. This may be a time-consuming process: although the patient lost only 60% of his small bowel and has adequate intestinal surface area for absorption, he did lose his ileocecal valve, which may alter intestinal transit time. He can be maintained by fat-containing peripheral vein infusions, although he is slightly obese and accessible veins in his arms are difficult to find. Because of the extended time that will probably be required to support this man, I would insert a central venous catheter for infusion of a fat-containing parenteral diet. Alternately, some nutrition units would use peripheral vein infusions initially and implant a silastic catheter which enters the subclavian vein and is tunneled subcutaneously to exit on the midchest (Broviac catheter). This catheter would provide long-term access for parenteral nutritional support and possibly allow the patient to feed himself by the intravenous route at home. Initially, albumin should be added to the infusate to restore colloid osmotic pressure and aid resolution of the edema, which may contribute to gastrointestinal dysfunction. When parenteral nutritional support is achieved and the edema has cleared, small volumes of a dilute chemically defined diet should be fed. If tolerated, volume and tonicity can be increased gradually. Take

your time; the transition period to achieve successful enteral feedings may take months, but with time the patient can be gradually converted to regular food and fed a high-carbohydrate, low-fat diet.

(11)   Supplement vitamins, minerals, and fat: When converted to an oral diet, the patient will require intermittent intramuscular administration of B_{12} and possibly folic acid. In addition, potassium, calcium, magnesium, and vitamin D supplements may be required. These requirements can be monitored by periodic determinations of blood concentrations.

Index